Plague Among the Magnolias

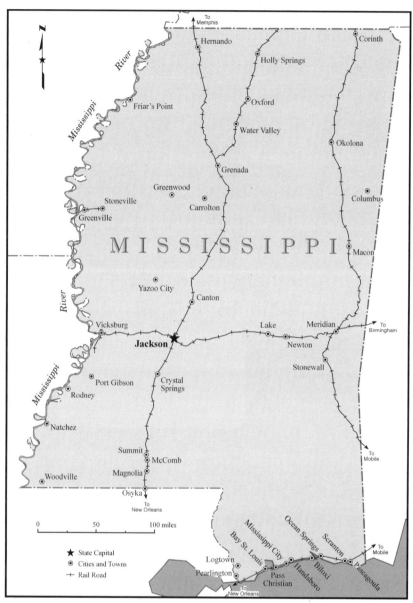

Mississippi in 1878, including towns and cities most affected by the yellow fever epidemic.

Plague Among the Magnolias

The 1878 Yellow Fever Epidemic in Mississippi

DEANNE STEPHENS NUWER

THE UNIVERSITY OF ALABAMA PRESS

Tuscaloosa

Typeface: Granjon

∞

The paper on which this book is printed meets the minimum requirements of
American National Standard for Information Sciences-Permanence of Paper for Printed
Library Materials, ANSI Z39.48-1984.

Library of Congress Cataloging-in-Publication Data

Nuwer, Deanne.
Plague among the magnolias : the 1878 yellow fever epidemic in Mississippi /
Deanne Stephens Nuwer.
p. ; cm.
Includes bibliographical references and index.
ISBN 978-0-8173-1653-2 (cloth : alk. paper) — ISBN 978-0-8173-8244-5 (e-book)
1. Yellow fever—Mississippi—History—19th century. I. Title.
[DNLM: 1. Yellow Fever—history—Mississippi. 2. Disease Outbreaks—history—
Mississippi. 3. History, 19th Century—Mississippi. 4. Public Health Practice—
history—Mississippi. WC 532 N989p 2009]
RC211.M7N89 2009
614.5′4109762—dc22

2008051232

Thank you to Dave, Rachel, and Amelia for their unending support. Special thanks
to Phyllis Jestice, William K. Scarborough, Bradley Bond, and Chuck Bolton for their
perceptive manuscript suggestions. Any remaining errors are my own.

Contents

List of Illustrations   vii

Preface   ix

1. Mississippi in the 1870s   1

2. Yellow Fever's Causes, Symptoms, and Treatments   6

3. The Fever Arrives   19

4. Responses to Yellow Fever   48

5. The Human Suffering   73

6. Mississippi and the Affirmation of Antebellum Values   89

7. Yellow Fever Departs   109

8. Conclusion   126

Notes   137

A Note on Resources   167

Bibliography   171

Index   185

Illustrations

MAP

Mississippi in 1878   frontispiece

TABLES

1. Leflore County congressional elections turnout, 1877 and 1878   43

2. Reported yellow fever cases and deaths in Mississippi in 1878   117

3. Relief aid received in Mississippi locales in 1878   121

4. Yellow fever cases and deaths in the United States
during the 1878 epidemic   128

5. Cotton production in Mississippi, 1877–1879:
Acreage, production, and yield   133

Preface

"In Memory of My Entire Family," reads the epitaph. The words are barely visible under the carpet of lichens covering a family monument hidden in overgrown bushes. This obscure reminder is all that remains of Beechland, Mississippi, a community that once existed near Vicksburg. Yellow fever ravaged Beechland and the rest of Mississippi in 1878, destroying lives, families, and even whole towns. That year's epidemic was the worst natural disaster nineteenth-century Mississippians experienced, and many of the state's towns and families never recovered.[1]

For example, the Featherstuns were a large family who lived in the Beechland community. Rev. F. M. Featherstun was a man of "noble" and "generous impulses" who, upon hearing news of the yellow fever outbreak, volunteered to minister to the sick. However, his own family subsequently fell ill, and by October 18, 1878, only two of eleven family members survived. Among the dead were Mary, age forty-eight; Wesley, nineteen; Abbie, sixteen; Willie, twelve; and Laura, ten. These victims were members of Featherstun's immediate family, but also residing at his home during the dire yellow fever days were his daughter-in-law, Laura; her sister, Abby Rundell; a son-in-law, W. B. Cleland; and Featherstun's four-week-old grandchild, Bobie. All of them died within a few days of one another during the epidemic. Only Featherstun and one daughter, Irene, the mother of Bobie, survived the scourge. The pastor erected a poignant monument in memory of his family. The Featherstuns, unfortunately, were not an unusual case in the 1878 yellow fever epidemic.[2]

Yellow fever struck Mississippi in July 1878 and maintained its grip until the end of November, testing the resolve of its citizens and the power of its newly created state board of health. Multitudes of Mississippians attempted to flee from the dreaded contagion. Thousands more died throughout the summer and fall months, accounting for more than 25 percent of the national yellow fever deaths in that year.

This study addresses the epidemic as it played out in Mississippi, revealing a populace fraught with frustrations and economic problems as citizens fought to survive yellow fever. It also outlines grassroots efforts by the state's citizens to combat the scourge. Through these efforts, Mississippi's public health care system ultimately took shape, grounded in a tradition of local organizations protecting citizens from health threats and taking responsibility for marshaling resources. A micro-study of Mississippi in this epidemic is useful because it reveals one more post-Reconstruction southern state adopting a new attitude about its place in the national agenda of health care when confronted with overwhelming demands. Even though Mississippi had a history of health care organizations and laws, the 1878 epidemic crystallized the need for the state to enter a more advanced stage of health care. After 1878, both Mississippi and yellow fever entered new historic periods: the former struggled with its place on the national stage, and scientists began the conquest of the latter.

Before the beginning of the nineteenth century, while Mississippi was still a United States territory, yellow fever and other contagious diseases were serious threats. In 1799, lawmakers prohibited any vessel or immigrant with a contagious disease such as yellow fever or smallpox from entering Mississippi. In 1803 and 1807 the territorial government strengthened the original law to include a fine of two thousand dollars or twelve months in prison for anyone who willfully brought a contagious disease into the territory. In 1817, the year Mississippi became a state, Natchez, a steamboat stop on the Mississippi River, organized the first city board of health, with five commissioners of health, including a police officer, appointed by the governor. This board established a quarantine station at Bacon's Landing, two miles below Natchez, to protect it from contagious diseases that might be harbored aboard the vessels steaming up and down the Mississippi. Thereafter, the 1857 Mississippi Law Code empowered other towns to pass regulations and adopt measures to prevent the introduction or spread of yellow fever and other diseases. From 1857 to 1876, no new sanitation or health laws were passed, even though the state medical association was organized in 1869. However, on March 24, 1876, the three coastal counties, Jackson, Harrison, and Hancock, created a coastal board of health to guard against yellow fever and to organize quarantine stations in each county. Each county was then authorized in 1877 to establish a board of health to combat the influx of disease. By February of that year the legislature created the Mississippi State Board of Health to contend with health care issues in the state, particularly yellow fever.[3]

Yellow fever had plagued the state from colonial times. The earliest extant reference to the disease in the region involved Pierre LeMoyne, Sieur d'Iberville, and his two brothers, Antoine and Jean Baptiste LeMoyne Bienville. In February 1699 Iberville established the first permanent French settlement along the

Gulf Coast at Fort Maurepas, on the eastern extremity of Biloxi Bay, where the city of Ocean Springs, Mississippi, now stands. Santo Domingo, the capital of the Dominican Republic, was the supply base for the French settlement. Because of its Atlantic shipping contacts with fever-ridden Africa and the Caribbean archipelago, Santo Domingo was frequently subjected to outbreaks of yellow fever. Iberville learned that on August 22, 1701, his brother and then-governor of the Mississippi outpost, Antoine Lemoyne Sauvolle de la Villantry, had died—apparently of yellow fever—at the Ocean Springs fortification.[4] A supply ship from Santo Domingo had probably carried the fever to Mississippi. From that beginning until 1905, when the last yellow fever epidemic appeared, Mississippi settlers lived intimately with the fear of outbreaks. By the late nineteenth century they dreaded, yet expected, regular occurrences of "Yellow Jack," as the disease was known to contemporaries.[5]

This book argues that what made Mississippi's 1878 yellow fever epidemic different was the expanded role played by charities and local government agencies, all struggling to find expression in the postwar South. The newly formed state board of health could not offer much assistance, but it did keep valuable statistics and extend advice to stricken areas. Provisions and financial aid arrived from a wide variety of sources, both within Mississippi and without. The Fraternal Order of the Masons maintained excellent records of collected monies and subsequent disbursements. The Howard Association, a benevolent organization with roots in antebellum New Orleans, was instrumental in providing medical personnel and monetary aid throughout this epidemic. If not for these services and others, suffering would have been much greater in Mississippi.

The story of the Mississippi State Board of Health is one of frustration and powerlessness, as Mississippians resented government control even as they expected help from government agencies. As the death toll mounted throughout the epidemic, the state health board issued numerous circulars on disinfectants as well as the board's rules for recording yellow fever cases and deaths. The board's secretary, Wirt Johnston, reporting after the epidemic, addressed the organization's role when he informed Governor John Marshall Stone in 1879 that "Under the present laws we [still] stand as an advisory body only, without power to establish quarantine or law to enforce it, with no appropriation to put into operation, and none to sustain it." Consequently, "circulars, letters, telegrams, instructions and advice in every shape and form was [sic] forwarded to every local Board in the State during the 1879 epidemic," but no official power existed for it.[6] The situation must have been frustrating for Mississippi officials, for just next door the Louisiana State Board of Health was a vital institution that had been in existence since March 15, 1855. Louisiana's health board could establish quarantine stations and had expanded powers and duties as designated by the Louisiana legislature. Louisiana quarantines were not always consistent, but Mississippi's board of health had no quarantine power at all. Mississippi lagged behind its sister state in regard to organized health care from a government agency and in quarantine regulations as both states simultaneously experienced the epidemic.[7]

It would be satisfying to report that the Mississippi State Board of Health came of age with the 1878 epidemic, but matters were not so simple. Dr. Johnston's complaints to the governor about the health board's powerlessness fell on deaf ears. Nonetheless, the physician left a valuable record, continuing to collect data about yellow fever as long as the disease ran its course. He requested statistics and information concerning yellow fever case numbers, deaths, expenditures, and epidemiological history from stricken locales. And, of course, he persisted in issuing circulars.

The epidemic had far-reaching effects on relief organization in Mississippi. It affected towns throughout the state that historically had been fever-free, and there were efforts at quarantine, though these were not very well organized. Quarantine lines, often guarded with shotgun-wielding patrols, quickly strangled much-needed inter- and intrastate commerce. Officials at Columbus, Mississippi, actually guarded the banks of the Tombigbee River with artillery and had orders "to sink any boat hailing from the direction of Mobile [Alabama]."[8] Mass confusion and panic permeated Mississippi's towns throughout the 1878 fever months as news of the ever-widening swath of infection reached locales once considered safe from yellow fever. Historian of science Charles E. Rosenberg asserts that public officials are unenthusiastic to acknowledge an epidemic because it is viewed as a dangerous "intruder": "The stakes have always been high, for to admit the presence of an epidemic disease was to risk social dissolution."[9] Businesses and state resources deteriorate through epidemics; in Mississippi in 1878 this progressed to the point that, within weeks, residents required monetary aid and relief supplies, including federal assistance and donations from as far away as California, Canada, and France.

Mississippians were not the only ones who suffered in 1878. Other states, most notably Louisiana and Tennessee, endured the catastrophe as well, with casualties in the thousands.[10] The epidemic reached as far north as New York State. However, Mississippi's experience in the epidemic is revealing because state and local officials responded to the epidemic's devastation by constructing an infrastructure of civic organizations and establishing an atmosphere of readiness that ultimately led to the establishment of a public health movement in the state. As historian John Ellis notes in *Yellow Fever and Public Health in the New South,* the 1878 epidemic revealed the need for a public health movement in the South, a region then woefully lacking in health care opportunities for its citizens. Ellis's study focuses on only three cities: New Orleans, Memphis, and Atlanta. These three urban centers were important to the development of the public health system in the South since they experienced multiple yellow fever epidemics as well as outbreaks of other diseases. Moreover, historian John Duffy explores in *The Sanitarians: A History of American Public Health* the broad public health movement from colonial to modern times, yet fails to mention any of Mississippi's health care efforts or epidemics. An exploration of that state's experiences in the 1878 yellow fever epidemic will help to explain a movement that covered all regions, not just key urban areas. By the end of the epidemic, many Mississippians recognized that their economic success depended largely upon the state's ability to assimilate national agendas, including health care.

Understanding the political environment of Mississippi prior to the 1878 yellow fever epidemic is also important. The years preceding the epidemic offer a glimpse into a southern state shaped by ten years of political and economic strife that ultimately influenced its efforts to build national connections while still trying to maintain some antebellum values. The result was the creation of a "new" Mississippi that fused old social values with new sociopolitical realities. It has long been recognized that in political terms Mississippi Reconstruction ended with the implementation of the Democrats' 1875 First Mississippi Plan and subsequent 1876 state elections.[11] White "redemption" of the state from Republican control initiated a two-pronged political takeover. First, in 1875, white voters secured political dominance in five of the six Mississippi congressional districts; second, African Americans were stripped of their civil rights through legal channels with the Mississippi 1890 Constitution.[12]

The deepest dividing issue in Reconstruction was of course racial relations. The Reconstruction federal government of 1865 had taken strong measures ensuring rights to former slaves, but by 1878 Mississippi legislators had created regulatory measures against African Americans that ultimately became the basis for the Mississippi Black Code. Even though African-American men were allowed to own property and initiate legal actions in court under this code, they were denied the right to testify against whites, serve on juries, join state militias, or vote.[13]

Poverty was also a factor in preventing the development of an effective government agency to cope with yellow fever. Economically, Reconstruction-era Mississippians continued to rely upon cotton as a staple crop to the exclusion of other agricultural commodities such as grains. When the cotton market fell in 1867, Mississippians found themselves saddled with debt, unable to repay loans. Citizens' delinquent tax bills also resulted in thousands of acres defaulting to the state. Land prices plummeted as debts skyrocketed. During this stressful time, the Freedmen's Bureau and some planters distributed provisions to the needy.[14]

Perhaps the most lasting legacy of Reconstruction still visible in 1878 was a deep suspicion of government interference as a threat to political rights and individual liberties. In 1867 the federal government had disenfranchised much of the white population—while giving the vote to male former slaves. By 1878 Mississippi Democrats had regained control, largely thanks to their ability to tap white southerners' outrage over being subordinated. They emphasized tradition, paternalism, self-reliance, and independence. This hegemony represented the antebellum South, including a nonchalant attitude toward the law. In an effort to defeat the Mississippi constitution in 1868, which would have disenfranchised the majority of whites, night riders used violent acts of intimidation. According to historians, the Ku Klux Klan and similar organizations campaigned to halt the ratification of that constitution by the "Kuklux method."[15] The threat of economic reprisals and violence helped the Democrats achieve their goal. Mississippi whites defeated the 1868 Republican constitution. However, after protests of fraud and intimidation, Republicans still sought to implement it.

By 1875, the Mississippi Plan to restore control to the Democratic Party had succeeded. By 1876, conservative Democrats regained control of the state legislature, and John Marshall Stone became the Democratic governor with a clear brief not to infringe on white Mississippians' right to self-determination. The 1878 epidemic, however, would teach the Mississippi Democrats that independence could only go so far. Regardless of their political agenda, some Democrats came to understand that the state would have to enter into a new era of health care, since the disaster had been too complex for them to manage independently. Mississippi had been unprepared and unable to care for its stricken citizens. By the Democrats' subsequent actions, the state's leadership acknowledged that Mississippi had to engage in and be a part of the national political and economic process, thereby ushering in an era that witnessed the state's entrance onto the national stage of public health.

By examining the rich collection of heretofore unexplored primary sources, it is possible to reconstruct the extraordinary efforts of ordinary Mississippians and others who provided aid and assistance during the epidemic. Family letters, doctors' accounts, and cemetery records reveal a day-to-day story of extreme duress. As one contemporary lamented, "There is no parallel in the history of yellow fever to the sufferings and mortality that has been upon us."[16] Newspaper sources, particularly the *Jackson Clarion* and the *Pascagoula Democrat-Star,* provide particularly valuable information.

A sociohistorical perspective of the yellow fever epidemic that clearly outlines the need for better and expanded health care efforts in Mississippi has yet to be explored fully. Previous studies such as Khaled J. Bloom's *The Mississippi Valley's Great Yellow Fever Epidemic of 1878,* John H. Ellis's *Yellow Fever and Public Health in the New South,* and Margaret Humphreys's *Yellow Fever and the South* only glanced at the state of Mississippi and did not adequately explore the narrative of its citizens who endured the epidemic. This work introduces the responses of Mississippians to this epidemic and reveals the state government's lack of preparedness and resources. More importantly, it shows how Mississippians recognized the need for better health care and began a public health movement in their state. In addition, this examination stresses the value of understanding regional cultures so that the impact of epidemics can be appreciated, particularly when an epidemic leads to the collapse of social restrictions. In this case, the breaking down of social boundaries between the North and South, and sometimes even between whites and African Americans, regardless of the ephemeral quality of those breakdowns, occurred as a result of social, economic, and political strains resulting from the epidemic. This analysis also illustrates that race shaped 1878 Mississippi as it structured people's lives; therefore, their responses were formed by racism and post-Reconstruction politics. Moreover, the study outlines the role played by national charities and other grassroots organizations that attempted to help Mississippians when the state was unable to do so. Thus, this story is significant not only in southern history but also for the broader understanding of American disaster relief and the emerging public health movement.

The study begins with a succinct historical look at Reconstruction in the state in order to provide a better understanding of post–Civil War Mississippi. It then progresses with an explanation of yellow fever etiology and accepted medical treatment of the time. Individual chapters then address quarantine efforts, charitable organizations, and the national public health movement. Throughout these chapters, the stories of Mississippians weave a narrative describing heroic efforts and horrific circumstances. At the conclusion, it is clear that Mississippi was on the precipice of stepping into a public health movement, already in progress, and that the 1878 yellow fever epidemic was the catalyst that motivated the state to take the final step.

Plague Among the Magnolias

I

Mississippi in the 1870s

A period of sifting and reckoning
> —Avery Odelle Craven, *Reconstruction: The Ending of the Civil War*

In the aftermath of the Civil War, Mississippians wrestled with political, economic, and social dislocation. The Civil War had destroyed the state's antebellum political and economic infrastructure, maintained previously by a carefully constructed patriarchal social order that valued self-reliance and independence. However, patriarchal social norms were not obliterated; they merely lay dormant, waiting for a chance to reemerge in the political sphere.

Mississippi was economically and politically devastated by the war. After Confederate forces surrendered east of the Mississippi on May 6, 1865, Mississippians inventoried the extent of destruction to town properties, railroads, and local governments. Vicksburg, especially, after enduring bombardment and a forty-seven-day siege in 1863, was economically wrecked. Other towns in the interior and along the Mississippi River also lay in ruin. Labor strife added further strain to the already broken economy. Roughly seventy-eight thousand Mississippians had fought in the war, nearly a third of them dying either of wounds or disease. The loss of white manpower combined with the emancipation of 437,303 African Americans in the state created an agricultural crisis, compounded by the fact that returning ex-Confederates arrived home too late for the 1865 planting season. Droves of freed African Americans migrated to the Delta in search of a livelihood, as others moved to more urban locales like Jackson seeking a new life.[1] Mississippi faced a period of transition with no blueprint for guidance.

Of course, losing the war did not mean that Mississippians' attitudes had suddenly been transformed. Slave labor had dominated the agricultural system, so whites tried to replicate that situation as closely as possible through sharecropping and crop-lien laws.[2] Since newly freed people had no money or means to earn cash, they worked for shares of a total harvest, with cotton being the acceptable crop. However, in years like 1866 and 1867, when cotton production fell below expectations, sharecroppers and landowners felt the pinch. Sharecroppers, especially, discovered themselves in a system of agricultural gridlock because they could rely only on plantation stores and other mercantiles for staples. They were captive consumers, victims of any price fluctuations. With little consumer savvy, they became mired in debt.[3] Both of these tactics, by 1867, secured the landowners' position at the pinnacle of the Mississippi socioeconomic pyramid and eventually relegated "croppers," both white and black, to the bottom.

Traditional patriarchal structures that militated against both African Americans and poor whites had to compete against imposed political realities, though. Partly as a result of frustrating economic situations but more certainly as a consequence of the first Reconstruction measures, passed in March 1867, a new political coalition emerged in Mississippi. African-American voters, already a majority, outnumbered whites even more after the new measures disenfranchised approximately 10 percent of ex-Confederates. Joining with the new black voters were poor whites, many of whom had been Unionists, and some wealthy former Whigs, who believed they could control the African-American voters. Northerners—Union soldiers who settled in the South and others who came later as teachers and church leaders—also allied with the African Americans.[4] They all participated in the new Mississippi government. African-American preachers, lawyers, and teachers from the North and Canada developed Loyal Leagues to help newly freed people become more politically educated and to provide them with social activities.[5]

In the national elections of 1868, however, most Mississippi Democrats rejected the Republican coalition and campaigned violently against its political efforts. The Democratic Party stressed traditionalism, paternalism, and self-determinism, embodying the core of antebellum values. However, terrorist tactics did not prevent a Republican majority in the Mississippi legislature and the election of Ulysses S. Grant as president. Mississippi Democrats did not accept the new political order. Their aggressive actions in the late 1860s presaged events of the 1870s. After all, the average southerner was likely to be offended by the Reconstruction agenda. Enfranchising former slaves and living under Republican rule were slaps in the face of societal traditions. Thus the sidelined Democrats of Mississippi fought for their threatened worldview. In the early 1870s they initiated a multi-pronged attack on African Americans to break the Republican control of state government by using intimidation, economic pressure, political recruitment, and acts of violence against black Mississippians.

In other words, white Mississippians had embraced the idea of political and social organization to achieve goals they considered desirable. But paradoxically, increased activism weakened the open, public actions of government. While many politicians were engaged in the war against Reconstruction, the government itself had to maintain a facade of legality.

Nothing illustrates this situation better than the state government's unequal treatment of racial incidents in the 1870s. The Meridian race riot in 1871 opened the volley of assaults. Several African-American men returned to Meridian on March 4 after attending a Republican political meeting in Jackson the previous day. While they gave a report on the rally to Meridian's African-American community, shouts warned the listening crowd about a fire at the home of William Sturgis, Meridian's Republican mayor. In the chaos that ensued, whites seized the opportunity to clamp down on the participants. Because white citizens perceived any political meeting held by African Americans as incendiary, they persuaded officials to arrest three black leaders and charge them with inciting a riot.[6] The arrests had nothing to do with the fire or their affiliation with the Republican Party; they hinged upon the racial strife already existing in the state and the public manner in which the three men had expressed their political views. At the trial approximately one week later, violence broke out in the courthouse, ending with the murder of the presiding Republican judge. Thereafter, order disintegrated and armed whites killed approximately thirty black Meridians. Mayor Sturgis received orders from the controlling whites to leave Mississippi within twenty-four hours. Democrats essentially ousted Republicans from control in Meridian with these violent events.[7] But, it is important to note two points: first, the Democrats involved were not acting through any government channel; and second, a political party was creating chaos rather than trying to prevent it.

The federal government tried to intervene, but the sheer fact of federal involvement merely compounded outrage. Mississippians—or at least those Mississippians who mattered politically—loathed the federal government. In an effort to thwart outbreaks such as the Meridian riot, the federal Enforcement Act of 1871 proscribed Ku Klux Klan activities, since many Republicans, including Governor James L. Alcorn, believed the Klan had instigated the events in Meridian. Certainly, though, the Klan was not the only organization terrorizing African Americans and Republicans. Other groups, such as the Knights of the White Camelia, the Sons of Midnight, and the White League, also interfered in the African Americans' civil and political rights.[8] The Klan was simply the most notorious. However, federal intervention did little to halt the violence in Mississippi; rather, it caused further disdain for the interfering government. Clashes between the races continued. Clara C. Young of Monroe County remembered that "De Yankees tried to git some of de men to vote, too, but not many did 'cause dey was scared of de Ku Kluxers. Dey would come at night all dressed up lak ghosts an' scare us all."[9] Terrorist tactics continued nonstop. In December 1874, local white militiamen killed approximately thirty-five African Americans in Vicksburg after a "tax-payers convention" of whites demanded the resignations of some city officials, including the sheriff, chancery clerk, and coroner.

Confrontations such as those in Monroe County, Meridian, and Vicksburg proved effective in setting the stage for the Democrats' plan in 1875. The Vicks-burg agenda of violence became the model for white conservatives across the state. In his study of Reconstruction, Vernon Lane Wharton quotes the *Vicks-burg Monitor*, which proclaimed: "The same tactics that saved Vicksburg will surely save the State, and no other will."[10] Disorder reigned in Mississippi as Democrats channeled traditional beliefs to end Republican rule.

The story of the fights to abolish Reconstruction in Mississippi and other southern states has been told elsewhere. Less considered, though, have been the lessons these efforts can teach us about ideas of government. Admittedly, fed-eral law blocked those seeking to return to the "good ol' days" from simple, straightforward political action. However, many of the Democratic politicians who emerged after 1876 had been trained in a system that actively opposed na-tional government. They encouraged "self-help" societies like the Klan and also encouraged individualism—at least among individuals of the "right" color and social class.

But by the election of 1876, no concealment was needed. Across the state, Claiborne, Kemper, Amite, Copiah, and Clay counties all reported public distur-bances during the election. Exercising violent tactics, Democrats used any and all means to ensure a win. In Aberdeen they trained a cannon on the polling place while a group of mounted Alabamians who supported the Mississippi Demo-crats' efforts patrolled on horses in front of the building to make certain that only like-minded men voted. In Columbus at least six fires blazed on election night as a warning that only Democrats would be allowed to participate in the next day's voting.[11]

The Democrats' efforts succeeded. With a thirty-thousand-majority vote across the state, Mississippi Democrats reported that "political emancipation" had occurred with the election of local officers and the majority of the legisla-ture. Sixty-two out of seventy-four counties saw the election of Democratic offi-cials.[12] Democrats then began sweeping out the state capital. Governor Adelbert Ames, forced to yield to Democratic pressure in the form of twenty-one articles of impeachment, resigned on March 29, 1876. The lieutenant governor and the superintendent of education, both African American, were also forced to leave.[13]

At the Democratic convention in August 1877, John Marshall Stone of Iuka received the nomination for governor and was later duly elected, beginning his term on January 10, 1878.[14] Stone had served as interim governor after Ames's resignation. He also appeared to be an ideal 1878 Democrat—an ex-Confederate who believed that Reconstruction had been just plain wrong.

When yellow fever broke out, Stone was thus governor of a state that had just undergone a massive political upheaval. John M. Stone had moved to Missis-sippi from Tennessee when he was twenty-five years old. Settling in Iuka, Tishomingo County, he first worked as a store clerk and later became a depot agent for the Memphis and Charleston Railroad. When the Civil War broke out he was among the first from his county to enlist.[15] Distinguishing himself at both Battles of Manassas and at Antietam, he was elected colonel of the Second Mississippi Regiment. Stone also saw action at Gettysburg, where he was wounded. After a medical furlough, he returned to combat and participated in the Battle of the Wilderness on May 6, 1864. In the last year of the war, Union forces captured him. Released after the war, he returned home a hero, and citizens of Iuka elected him mayor in 1866. After serving as mayor of Iuka and treasurer of Tishomingo County, he was elected to the Mississippi Senate in 1869 and again in 1873 before becoming governor.[16]

When yellow fever appeared in Mississippi in July 1878, the Democratic "redemption" process was well under way. However, pockets of Republican officeholders, both white and African American, remained in communities across the state, particularly in grassroots-level positions. The result was far-reaching distrust among the various levels of government and a great deal of confusion, both of which had the potential to hamper an effective response to the epidemic.

2

Yellow Fever's Causes, Symptoms, and Treatments

From slimy swamps and fathomless morasses
—James A. Martling, "The Yellow Fever—1878"

Two years after the Democrats had gained control of the Mississippi capital, one of the most severe yellow fever epidemics to hit the South occurred. The pestilence crossed all social and economic boundaries, adding to the chaos of the post–Civil War era to disrupt nineteenth-century life beyond imagination. Many Mississippians who lived through the 1878 epidemic left behind descriptions of their tribulations. Some who died during the epidemic are therefore remembered through the recollections of family members, friends, or neighbors and through their own words as revealed in personal letters and diaries. While terrible conditions also prevailed in many other states during the 1878 epidemic, the epidemic provides historians a window through which to view nineteenth-century Mississippians as they wrestled with economic hardship, racial tensions, sketchy medical knowledge, and ineffectual state relief efforts.

To comprehend the impact of the 1878 epidemic and the failure of efforts to control it, one must first understand the nature and symptoms of yellow fever, its various nineteenth-century medical treatments, and the modes of yellow fever transmission as understood by nineteenth-century Mississippians. Yellow fever, a tropical and subtropical disease caused by a virus, is also known as the saffron scourge, Yellow Jack, Bronze John, and the "yellow Tyrant of the tropics." In severe cases, renal failure and hematemesis, or "black vomit," are characteristic. Hematemesis occurs when bleeding takes place in the upper gastrointestinal tract and gastric acid alters the blood into the characteristic coffee-ground vomitus. Jaundice is typical, the effect of which gives the disease its name. Yellow fever is transmitted from person to person through the female *Aedes aegypti* mosquito.[1]

The exact origin of yellow fever is debated. Some historians earlier suggested that the disease originated in the Western Hemisphere, but in more modern times the accepted theory is that Europeans introduced yellow fever from Africa into the New World via commercial shipping along the African transatlantic trade routes. When Hernando de Soto explored the Mississippi region in the 1540s, yellow fever was unknown in North America. More than likely, the holds of Spanish slave-trading ships transported the disease to commercial markets in Mexico, the Caribbean, and then North America. Once yellow fever arrived in Mexico and the West Indies, it spread quickly, reaching Cuba by 1648.[2]

After yellow fever developed in the Gulf of Mexico region, it spread throughout North America along maritime and overland trade routes. The virus spread easily, carried onto ships by the ever-present *A. aegypti* mosquitoes and by viremic individuals or those already infected with the disease. This species of mosquito readily adapted to environments created by Europeans, since it breeds well in stagnant or slow-moving water such as that found in water casks, holds of ships, and cisterns. The mosquito could remain on board a ship for months, feeding on and reinfecting crews and travelers.[3]

Wherever it occurred, yellow fever followed a particular pattern. For transmission to occur, the female *A. aegypti* must feed on the blood of an infected individual within three to six days after that person contracts the disease. During those few days, the virus is most concentrated in the blood of the host, but the victim may or may not exhibit any symptoms of the disease. Any *A. aegypti* mosquito that feeds upon the blood of an infected person in that time frame then also becomes a vector of the yellow fever virus. It takes approximately two weeks for the ingested virus to reach the mosquito's salivary glands so that she is able to inject the virus while taking a blood meal. Obviously, the cycle could continue for a long time aboard a ship if viremic persons were aboard. Ships could then transport the adult and larval mosquitoes throughout a region, including the Mississippi coast. In addition, the insects, in cooler weather especially, can rest on a person's clothing or other surfaces and be disseminated in that manner. Therefore, in the 1878 epidemic, people unknowingly spread yellow fever as viremic individuals or as mosquito carriers when they fled from epidemic areas to safer, fever-free regions. Since the yellow fever virus cannot exist independently of a host, it must multiply both in vertebrates, such as monkeys and humans, and in arthropods, such as mosquitoes. However, in a classic urban epidemic, humans and *A. aegypti* are interdependent organisms.[4]

The course of yellow fever can be horrific, as described by many throughout the eighteenth and nineteenth centuries. Once "bitten" by the *A. aegypti* vector, the victim usually shows symptoms of the illness within four days. The first symptoms to appear are a high fever, flushed face, bloodshot eyes, and chills. The victim's temperature often soars to between 102 and 104 degrees, with temperatures recorded as high as 111 degrees.[5] The victim's fever then drops, and an appearance of general health and improvement ensues. Despite this appearance, the disease continues to make its way through the victim's body. Shortly after the lull of symptoms, the skin begins to turn lemon yellow as a result of dramatic jaundice, and other symptoms, such as nausea, constipation, headache, and often severe muscular pains in the legs and back, also appear. At this stage, bleeding begins in the mucous membranes, gums, and in the stomach in the more acute cases.

Another common term for yellow fever, "black vomit," derives from the regurgitation of partially digested blood. According to one nineteenth-century physician, "black vomit is combined with profuse intestinal hemorrhages, with bleeding from the nose, the mouth and the gums."[6] Some observers recorded yellow fever victims who did not discharge black vomit, but as one eyewitness of the disease noted in 1849, these victims merely "bled from various parts before or after death."[7] Even though the victims did not discharge "black vomit," they discharged blood of the mucous membranes from other orifices. As one Nashville doctor reported in 1878: "I remember upon one occasion being saved from a baptism of black vomit by my venerable friend and co-laborer, . . . who, as I was leaning intently over a patient seized me suddenly by the arm and drew me back from the bed just a moment before the ejection was made almost to the top of the musquito [sic] bar."[8] The mosquito bar held the mosquito netting that draped over the victim's bed, so the height of the bar could easily have been six or more feet. Mosquito netting provided protection from the incessant buzzing and biting of the insects; it was not used at this time as a preventive measure. Black vomit is usually the harbinger of death in yellow fever patients, occurring within the last two days of the victim's life. The effluent resembled coffee grounds, and according to contemporary observers, the patient exerted little physical effort in the vomiting process.[9]

In their descriptions of the disease's progression, nineteenth-century physicians recorded two distinct hemorrhaging symptoms associated with yellow fever. The first was a passive hemorrhage, as in bruising. This resulted from the death of blood corpuscles and the destruction of tissue when the "interior walls of . . . some of the larger veins were gone, giving the surface something of the appearance of the tracks which earthworms make in moist ground."[10] The second kind was the bleeding that occurred in the upper digestive tract and mucous membranes and the consequential vomiting of semidigested blood, ejected with little effort and "thrown considerable distance."[11] Modern medical knowledge explains that both types of hemorrhages resulted from disintegrated blood when the yellow fever virus destroyed the blood corpuscles.

Today's physicians know that damage to the liver, kidneys, and heart also occurs as yellow fever travels throughout the victim. Dissections of victims' bodies by nineteenth-century doctors revealed that the liver and spleen were greatly enlarged. However, nineteenth-century doctors did not list another symptom, leukopenia, which involves a low number of circulating white blood cells and a low production of white blood cells within the bone marrow. Today it is recognized that in the most severe yellow fever cases, death generally results from renal failure, heart failure, toxemia, and internal infection. Many nineteenth-century physicians reported albuminous urine or complete renal failure. Because of the low white blood cell count, the victim's body did not fight the disease adequately. Many mild infections of yellow fever, however, remained undiagnosed in the nineteenth century because of the disease's generally vague symptoms at the onset. Past and present, the majority of patients begin to recover within a week or two after contracting the disease. A full convalescence requires complete bed rest and stringent nursing care, often for several weeks.[12] Obviously, nineteenth-century recuperation was vastly different from modern health care in its quality and therapeutics. Even people of the nineteenth century, though, recognized that this disease left its victims helpless to care for themselves, thus necessitating help ranging from nursing to provision of food. They also knew that yellow fever could infect entire families, making external aid vital for survival.

The first outside recourse was the physician, but physicians could give only limited help, since they understood neither the disease nor how to treat it. Throughout the nineteenth century, major conflicting medicinal philosophies existed regarding how to treat diseases. The allopathic, homeopathic, and physio-medical approaches were often diametrically opposed. These approaches had advocates in Mississippi during the 1878 yellow fever epidemic, but as Earnest Hardenstein, a Vicksburg homeopathic physician, wrote that year, "There is not harmony of thought or action, no general law which seems to guide them [physicians], like a fixed star, through the darkness of theory and conjecture."[13]

Allopaths, or traditional physicians, often tried "heroic" methods of treatment to produce effects different from the symptoms of the disease being treated, and the prescriptives were usually in massive doses. Allopathy was more popular in the 1853 epidemic, but it still had its adherents in the 1878 visitation. One such physician was a Dr. Gibson of the Yazoo City region. Gibson kept a detailed prescription book that he used in treating everything from abscesses to warts. In his book he listed eighteen prescriptions for yellow fever. One of these medications mixed a solution of arsenic, quinine sulphate, and cherry laurel water with a few drops of sulphuric acid to dissolve the quinine.[14] The yellow fever patient took a teaspoonful of this mixture after meals. However, the most interesting therapeutic listed by Gibson was entitled "To Keep Mosquitoes away." The recipe called for three parts olive oil, two parts pennyroyal, one part glycerin, and one part ammonia. Gibson admonished that the mixture needed "to be well shaken when used, [and] be carefull [sic] about getting into eyes." European pennyroyal has a strong odor offensive to insects and is poisonous. Gibson's repellent recipe probably kept mosquitoes away, but his other prescriptions would not have cured yellow fever. Regardless of his knowledge of medicinal plants, Gibson's remedies exemplify the medical ignorance concerning yellow fever and its etiology, a characteristic common to both physicians and the general public in 1878.[15]

Homeopaths advocated a different medical approach to treatment. Samuel Christian Hahnemann (1755–1843), a German physician who had lost faith in allopathic medical practices, created and guided homeopathy in the early part of the nineteenth century. His discontent with and subsequent rebellion against traditional medicine criticized the generally accepted practices of massive enemas, violent laxatives, and excessive dosages of medicines. Hahnemann set forth his tenets of homeopathy in *Organon of Rational Healing* (1810). Two principles defined homeopathy: the doctrine of infinitesimal dosages and the doctrine of *similia similibus curantur,* or "like cures like." Both tenets stressed the importance of using minute quantities of medicines to produce results. According to the doctrine of similars, any drug that produces symptoms in a healthy person should help to cure a sick one. Therefore, once those drugs prove to be effective, the homeopathic physicians prescribes small dosages of them. The greatest service to the patient, according to Hahnemann, is to use the smallest amount of pharmaceuticals needed to treat a disease.[16]

As Hahnemann's philosophy gained popularity in the United States, homeopaths organized the American Institute of Homeopathy in 1844. Hahnemann Medical College, an American homeopathic school providing training for future physicians studying this approach, opened in 1848 in Philadelphia. Homeopathy's popularity increased greatly, and by the 1890s more than twenty such colleges existed throughout the United States. The closest homeopathic institution to Mississippi was the Southwestern Homeopathic Medical College in Louisville, which may have attracted Mississippi medical students prior to 1878.[17]

Perhaps because a homeopathic medical school was nearby or because of the growing popularity and effectiveness of this newer approach, sixteen Mississippi physicians were practicing homeopathy in 1878, including two in Natchez and eight in Vicksburg.[18] It is most likely because of their close relationship with New Orleans that Vicksburg and Natchez had more homeopathic practitioners than other locales in Mississippi. In 1878, New Orleans listed twelve homeopathic physicians and an active homeopathic professional organization. The Mississippi River provided a communication link for medical exchange and news among the ports of Natchez, Vicksburg, and New Orleans.[19]

One of the best-known of Mississippi's homeopaths was Vicksburg's A. O. H. Hardenstein, the father of Dr. Earnest Hardenstein. The elder Hardenstein had practiced medicine for fifty years before he compiled an outline of his methods for healing yellow fever in "A Treatise on the Disease, and a Concise Method of Treatment." The work explained yellow fever's etiology and outlined homeopathic remedies. It also includes homeopathic therapies and philosophies for a multitude of ailments. Hardenstein adamantly believed that homeopaths should have a "faith in the grand law of Hahnemann" and "not use leeches, practice bloodletting, blistering or put the patient in an icebox." These treatments, according to Hardenstein, were "needless cruelty." He further asserted that even self-treatment through homeopathy will "give far better results then [sic] the most accomplished old school doctor [allopath] can show, with his purgatives, blisters, plasters, quinine, calomel, cupping, leeching, refrigerating process, etc."[20]

The older Hardenstein consulted a New York insurance company's statistical chart to illustrate homeopathy's benefits. He showed that the insurance company charged lower rates to patrons who practiced homeopathy. According to Hardenstein's interpretation of this company's statistics, the patients of allopaths had a death rate three times greater than that of the patients of homeopaths. He insisted that insurance companies always carefully calculated their risks; therefore, since this particular New York establishment discovered that patrons treated by allopaths during an epidemic died in a ratio of three to one over those treated by homeopaths, the company changed its rates to reflect that risk. Hardenstein ended his argument for the benefits of homeopathy by openly challenging, "Can this be disputed?"[21]

Reporting on the 1878 yellow fever epidemic, the Homeopathic Yellow Fever Commission concurred with Hardenstein. He stated that their published report revealed that "the Homeopaths showed themselves faithful students and disciples of nature, not only in their judicious use of these things [materia medica], but in their uniform advocacy of plenty of fresh air, light covering, cold water, and an abstinence from all debilitation and perturbating treatment, in which they had often to contend with the violent prejudice of the people, long trained in the false doctrines of the old system." The commission concluded that only the homeopaths acted in similarity of practice "as if they worked together and kept step to the music of some great guiding law."[22]

Like the homeopaths and allopaths, the physio-medical adherents had their roots in an earlier group, the botanico-medical movement. Founded by Samuel Thomson in the late 1700s as an alternative to orthodox approaches, the botanico-medical approach was based on Thomson's theory that vegetable materia medica was more effective than the prescriptions of the medical establishment of the time.

Thomson grew up in the wilderness of New Hampshire and at an early age exhibited a curiosity about the native plants. He was influenced by an elderly woman named Benton, who took an interest in teaching him local plant lore.

She was the only person in the region who acted as a physician for the inhabitants, using herbs and roots as pharmaceuticals. Thomson walked with her in the woods and meadows while she instructed him about the indigenous plants and their effects on the human body.[23] Early America had many who used indigenous plants to concoct home remedies. For Thomson later to advocate such a system of medical treatment was not unusual; however, his innovative approach in patenting his remedies was out of the ordinary because previously, physicians who utilized herbal remedies often acted independently.[24]

Thomson patented his botanico-medical system over three different years, and his therapeutics grew in popularity. He based his system on the belief that a balance must be maintained with his *materia medica* between the four elements that constitute all bodies—earth, air, fire, and water. "Earth and water constitute the solids, and air and fire, or heat, are the cause of life and motion," he wrote. "Cold, or lessening the power of heat, is the cause of all disease . . . a state of perfect health arises from a due balance or temperature of the four elements."[25] By the 1830s, "Thomson's Patent" to maintain good health became the medical choice of many Americans seeking alternative medical treatments. Followers of his unorthodox medical system organized themselves into Friendly Botanic Societies, holding seven conventions from 1832 to 1838 and calling their meetings the United States Botanic Conventions.[26]

The Thomsonian movement, however, fractured over therapeutics and sales. During the 1850s and 1860s, numerous medical movements spun around Thomsonianism, so that by the 1878 yellow fever epidemic, the original movement had evolved into the botanics. These "irregulars" were particularly popular in the South. One 1873 list of physicians in Mississippi includes 646 regular physicians (allopaths), 13 homeopaths, and 49 irregulars (mostly botanics). It is reasonable to assume that just five years later, the number of botanics practicing in Mississippi during the yellow fever epidemic would not have changed dramatically; therefore, they would have outnumbered homeopaths. John S. Haller Jr. writes, "In most instances, their [the allopaths] chief sectarian rivals were the homeopaths, except in the South, where the numbers of miscellaneous practitioners (many of them holdovers from Thomsonianism) continued to vie even with the regulars."[27]

Allopaths, homeopaths, and botanics used pharmaceuticals to produce far different results in their yellow fever patients. The homeopaths' guiding law was the caveat against large doses of medicines, whereas allopaths experimented with varying amounts of therapeutics, searching for a yellow fever panacea. Botanics attempted to control disease through enemas, syrups, teas, and other *medica materia*. All schools of medical theory, however, encountered great trouble in treating symptoms at the onset of yellow fever. No school was successful in treating patients during the initial stages of the disease. Moreover, physicians had no particular mandated treatments from any board of health. The treatment people got depended upon geographical accident, word of mouth, or successful advertising.

Of all of the early yellow fever symptoms, high fever was the most challenging for a physician. Adherents of all schools of thought produced voluminous examples of treatments during this critical first stage. The Homeopathic Yellow Fever Commission best illustrated the difficulty in treating the high fever: "The great therapeutic question of the first stage is how to reduce the extreme high temperature, which, if long continued, will inevitably destroy the integrity of the blood and arrest the processes of nutrition in the molecules of every organ of the body."[28]

Physicians' opinions and remedies for treating the high fever associated with the beginning of yellow fever appeared in numerous professional journals, including the *Louisville Medical News*. Medical recommendations for treating the first stage of the disease varied. One South Carolina physician believed the patient should "at the very inception of the attack" have cold sponges applied to the head, hands, and arms, followed by fifteen to twenty-five grains of calomel, "with the same of quinine." The purgative calomel, also known as mercurous chloride, cleansed the gastrointestinal tract, while quinine supposedly reduced inflammation or fever and killed invading organisms in the body. Generally, homeopaths did not use calomel and quinine in their recommended treatments, recognizing that quinine affected a patient's hearing adversely and that calomel caused profuse vomiting. Additionally, the Charleston physician recommended that one-eighth to one-twelfth of a grain of morphine be administered two or three times a day while the patient's feet were in a hot mustard bath and a mustard plaster covered his or her abdomen. Dr. John L. Clark of Hickman, Kentucky, argued that a patient in the febrile stage of the disease should be covered with heavy blankets in a closed room or given hot teas, not calomel or quinine. "Such treatment," stated Clark, "is a relic of the barbarous practice of a quarter of a century ago."[29]

In 1878, Dr. R. W. Mitchell of Memphis outlined a somewhat different treatment for the initial stage of yellow fever. Mitchell stated that if a patient's temperature rose above 102 degrees, sponging with equal amounts of whiskey and water proved effective, as well as administering ten grains of quinine twice within the first twenty-four hours. He also insisted that his patients be absolutely quiet in "body and mind" during this first stage: "the world closes upon the patient until I turn him loose; he sees nothing, hears nothing, and remains perfectly quiet in bed."[30] Mitchell appears to have taken medical isolation to a new height in his treatment methods.

Dr. A. O. H. Hardenstein agreed with the general sense of these treatments for his patients in Vicksburg. Hardenstein concurred that a well-ventilated room for yellow fever patients was therapeutic, but he warned against featherbeds, as they were too warm and had no "adaptability for a change of position." On the other hand, the Vicksburg homeopath did not agree with the calomel or quinine dosages and tortuous mustard plasters and baths. He and other homeopaths often suggested teas, such as black, watermelon, or orange leaf, as medicines, as they helped to rehydrate the patient. Ultimately, however, Hardenstein admitted that there "is no more difficult task on earth than waiting on a yellow fever case."[31] Regardless of that caveat, homeopathy was a popular treatment option, perhaps because of its appeal to traditional self-reliance.

During the 1878 epidemic, the difficulty in treating yellow fever patients did not deter doctors—allopathic, homeopathic, or botanic—from trying a variety of methods to assuage the symptoms of the disease. Contemporary medical journals are filled with physicians' testimonials regarding the best and most successful treatments. For instance, Dr. J. Livingston of New Orleans wrote an explanation and remedy for yellow fever using "the application of natural law." He proposed that the fever stage could be ameliorated in a very short time if the physician bathed the yellow fever patient in ammonia or spirits of hartshorn for two or three hours. According to Livingston, the natural law of evaporation worked best with either of these two solutions to cool the patient. Although his allopathic treatment was not generally accepted by other doctors, Livingston believed it would appeal to the nonmedical public, vowing, "My theory is plain remedy, cheap and always at hand, and if it does not cure, it can not kill." However, the oil of the hartshorn plant irritates skin and mucous membranes and may cause blistering. Bathing in this certainly could be hazardous, as could the ammonia mixture.[32]

Some physicians experimented with various medicines in treating yellow fever and then presented their findings in professional medical publications. Sundry yellow fever prescriptions and mortality rates during disease months appeared in these journals. For example, Dr. W. H. Falls of Cincinnati stated that he tried a scarlet fever prescription on one yellow fever patient because a colleague had had "great success" with it while treating that disease. He also administered massive doses of calomel in his trial-by-error treatments. Of the five patients whom Falls describes in this article, four received calomel, and all four of those patients died. The extreme amount of calomel probably exacerbated the dehydration experienced because of continuous vomiting. Not to be discouraged, Falls stated that he would try salicylate of soda on future yellow fever patients as a "further trial."[33]

Medical approaches varied greatly. Botanics promoted the use of tonics and syrups containing natural ingredients such as bayberry and sassafras root, combined often with sweating. Homeopaths advocated the provision of nursing care and making the patient as comfortable as possible. Management of the disease should be supportive and help to alleviate major symptoms, such as headache and vomiting. Complete bed rest was also important, as was the correction of fluid imbalances caused by vomiting, sweating, and dehydration in order to treat a patient successfully. Homeopaths and physio-medicals emphasized these treatments, whereas allopaths did not.

In 1878, homeopaths had established a niche for themselves in the Mississippi medical community despite unfavorable reviews earlier from the traditional practitioners. After orthodox physicians formed the American Medical Association in 1847, that organization and the American Institute of Homeopathy would be at odds with one another until well into the twentieth century. However, homeopathy continued to grow in popularity, and during the 1878 yellow fever epidemic homeopaths provided some relief to their many patients, as did physiomedicals. The rigorous and often polypharmaceutical treatments of allopaths contrasted sharply with the more benign homeopathic and botanic treatments. As a result, homeopathy often appealed to the middle and upper classes, which were better informed and therefore more aware of alternative medical options. These same people were probably the social leaders of their communities, since they enjoyed a higher economic class.[34] Physio-medicals, on the other hand, appealed to the common folks, the "root and herb" people. As stated in the *American Journal of Pharmacy,* "the idea that each individual head of a family should in medicine, as in religion and politics, think and act for himself, presented so inviting an aspect to the yeomen of this land, that his [Thomson's] medical system was adopted as a revelation."[35]

Schools of medical thought endorsed a variety of theories to explain how yellow fever spread. Although these explanations may appear somewhat primitive and inadequate in the light of modern medical knowledge, contemporaries of the 1878 epidemic believed in and practiced the medical theories of the era. Three major explanations concerning the transmission of yellow fever existed: miasmic theory, fomite theory, and social causation theory.

According to the miasmic theory, yellow fever was caused by foul exhalations from putrefying animal or vegetable matter. By 1878 the medical community did not accept this explanation as widely as it once had, because the germ theory had been introduced since the 1853 epidemic. However, "bad air" nevertheless appeared as a cause in some publications, and the general public accepted this theory during the 1878 epidemic. The public's belief in this theory is important in social terms, as officials in various locales tried various cleanup schemes to rid the community of its foul air. Miasmic theory explains that exhalations from such items as animal carcasses, rotting oysters in cellars, hides in ships or on wharves, bacon, exposed graves, rotten corn, stagnant water, and mud and filth in shoal harbors (including slimy riverbanks) cause subtle, deleterious gases. These exhalations from putrefying animal and vegetable matter entered the victim's body through the lungs, filtered into the vital organs, and then produced disease. Many people also regarded general city filth in sewers as a potential miasmic producer. Supposedly, however, miasmas ceased when the temperature dropped below 32 degrees Fahrenheit.[36]

The fomite theorists, by contrast, declared that objects that could absorb germs or upon which germs could adhere were the agents of transmission. Although the miasmic theory had numerous advocates, many also contended that fomites were the cause of yellow fever, and their advocacy explains the intense fumigation processes that locales introduced—particularly in shipping regions of Mississippi—as the epidemic progressed through the state. The adherents of this school stated that noxious discharges from the stomach, bowels, skin, and even the breath of a person infected with yellow fever were able to stick to furniture or be absorbed by clothing and carpets. One contemporary physician wrote that yellow fever "is transmissible, communicable, and portable. You can smell it, and almost taste it," adding, "Whether a germ or not I cannot say, but it is tangible. . . . It will cling to the clothes, for I have tested it thoroughly by the sense of smell. . . . It has a peculiar and not a very disagreeable odor."[37] Supporters of this theory believed that fomites could even penetrate walls and holds of ships, thus contaminating other people. To thwart the spread of fomites, their means of transport, such as trains, had to be controlled as they traveled around the region. For example, Andrew Kilpatrick opined in 1844 that "if an epidemic should prevail in New Orleans, [and] the [train] cars here were permitted to run, there would be no difficulty in the transmission of fomites," as they could be carried throughout the city. As yellow fever spread throughout Mississippi in 1878, little doubt remained as to the portability of the disease.[38] It was only the exact cause that remained the mystery. Disinfectants, applied through fumigation processes, supposedly rendered the noxious dischargers or "germs" ineffectual.[39]

The social causation theory reflected the strict code of morals that generally governed society in the late nineteenth century. Social ethicists did not tolerate immorality, and social behavior was inflexible for many in certain socioeconomic strata. As an example of the strong moral code prevalent during this time, J. P. Dromgoole wrote in 1878 concerning yellow fever that "in no disease is a sound mind in a sound body more important." He stressed upright living and behavior to avoid contagion. A typical New Orleans doctor stated that yellow fever is "a mental, moral malady" and considered it a "consolidation of all the diseases through mental action or fear of death." Those who were careless in their moral and physical habits were supposedly the ones most likely to be afflicted with the fever. Therefore, proponents of this theory blamed African Americans, immigrants, and poorer people who lacked proper sanitation and personal hygiene for breeding and maintaining yellow fever "germs." Moreover, drunkenness, vice, debaucheries of any form, and even keeping late hours all contributed to the continuation of yellow fever, proponents of this theory claimed. It is not surprising that moral elitists blamed immigrants for contributing to the yellow fever epidemic as increasingly large numbers of immigrants from southern and eastern Europe poured into the United States. As these newcomers settled in cities like New Orleans, many of them brought with them foreign languages, odd clothing, and cultural mores unfamiliar to natives. Moreover, immigrants usually sought housing in less desirable urban areas because they lacked necessary resources and skills to afford better. Therefore, natives considered many immigrant neighborhoods seething ports of disease. Even though Mississippi did not experience the immigrant influx that other regions did, prejudice against immigrants mirrored the white stance toward African Americans in the state.[40] What the social causation theorists failed to recognize was that the "depraved" inhabitants lived in close proximity to the cesspools and stagnant water accumulations that were the breeding grounds of *A. aegypti,* as well as the docks and dwellings frequented by the infected yellow fever carriers.

The mode of yellow fever transmission was unknown, and no overarching explanation existed for the contagion's apparent randomness. Not until 1893 would Theobald Smith and Fred Lucius Kilbourne from the federal Bureau of Animal Industry demonstrate that ticks carried the pathogen for Texas fever in cattle. From that revelation, scientists would eventually conquer other diseases as they began to understand and unravel the life cycle of other devastating diseases such as yellow fever.[41] Until that time, state agencies were simply reacting to a crisis with little if any effective scientific grounding. Nevertheless, other states went further than Mississippi in using measures such as quarantines to limit yellow fever's ravages. Mississippi, with a paralyzed state government that had come into being through a gospel of independence and self-help, lacked both the will and the means for significant intervention. Instead, communities relied on local initiative, reverting to the grassroots level of self-governance typical of antebellum Mississippi in their attempts to explain the transmission of the disease.

This chapter has provided insight into the terror associated with yellow fever in the nineteenth century and the views of disease that were popular during that time. No one group held a monopoly on yellow fever treatment in 1878, even though all physicians acknowledged the contagiousness of the disease and suggested quarantines to keep it at bay. Regardless of the therapeutics touted and the transmission theories espoused by the physicians and citizens of 1878 Mississippi, their faith ultimately rested in the only cure that consistently provided positive results: temperatures below 32 degrees Fahrenheit. Even though they did not know that those temperatures were low enough to kill the mosquito vector and its larvae, local papers celebrated whenever temperatures reached the freezing point. An editor for the *Jackson Daily Bulletin* best summed this up when he wrote that "Dr. Jack Frost is the only yellow fever expert in whom the people have absolute confidence."[42]

3
The Fever Arrives

Prior to 1878, Mississippians had experienced numerous yellow fever epidemics. During those outbreaks, state and local agencies had opportunities to show how well they responded to citizens' needs, both real and perceived. The 1878 epidemic was by far the worst visitation, but earlier epidemics can provide a sense of antebellum occurrences for comparison to 1878. This chapter highlights the importance of economics, showing how costly quarantines could be for local businesses, and illustrates the problems that occurred because of a lack of uniform directions from an impotent state board of health. Thus it illuminates the tensions involved when individual liberty and the public welfare clashed in the 1878 yellow fever epidemic in Mississippi.

Mississippians feared and expected regular outbreaks of yellow fever. For all visitations of the disease, the fever season typically began in the summer months and ended with the first frost, usually in November. The severity and prevalence of each epidemic varied. The 1853 epidemic was particularly virulent, especially in Louisiana and along the Mississippi Gulf Coast.[1] Those who lived there along sludge-filled bayous as well as those on high, dry ground experienced yellow fever that year; no social class or economic standing protected individuals in this outbreak. As a result, approximately 10,000 New Orleanians out of 30,000 reported cases died in that epidemic. Contemporaries labeled the city the "Necropolis of the South" because of its case/mortality rate of roughly 33 percent. The city had a population of approximately 116,000 that year. The pestilence was equally devastating in Mississippi, although the state had no cities comparable in size to New Orleans. In Biloxi, one doctor recorded 111 deaths out of 533 reported cases in the 1853 epidemic, a fatality rate of approximately 21 percent. The population of that small coastal town was roughly 1,700, but its numbers had swelled to 6,000 as panic-stricken New Orleanians fled to the Mississippi Gulf Coast in an effort to escape the dire circumstances in their Louisiana city.[2]

Yellow fever epidemics required community effort, because, wherever the location, quarantine was the accepted way to deal with it. For example, in 1855 Louisiana legislators created the Louisiana State Board of Health, the first such board in the United States, in direct response to the horrific 1853 yellow fever epidemic. The board's primary function was to enforce quarantine regulations for the state by maintaining three ship-inspection stations on waterways leading into Louisiana—the Mississippi River, the Atchafalaya River, and the entrance to Lake Pontchartrain from the Gulf of Mexico (the Rigolets).[3] Quarantines became the standard containment procedure for communities throughout the South, especially after the Louisiana state board led the way.

In 1855, however, Mississippi did not follow as stringent a quarantine plan. It is useful to explore the reason for the differences between the two neighbor states. One reason was doubtless the much greater urbanization of Louisiana. Even the most casual observer could see that the great port of New Orleans imported disease as well as market goods. In addition, local government structures had managed to address events in Mississippi's 1853 epidemic without a state board of health. City authorities had declared and maintained quarantines for as long as yellow fever exhibited itself.

In some ways the situation was similar in 1878. The mode of transmission was still unknown, and quarantines remained the normal way of dealing with yellow fever outbreaks. However, the political climate in the 1878 epidemic differentiated it from the 1853 outbreak. The big question in 1878 was whether Reconstruction had wrecked the paternalistic infrastructure of antebellum southerners or merely driven it underground. How would the Redeemers respond in this situation?

As bad as the 1853 epidemic was, it was eclipsed by the 1878 outbreak in its geographic spread and in its mortality rate. Susan Alexander Simpson of Pensacola wrote to her daughter, Kate Simpson, on August 20, 1878, that she was unable to leave Florida because yellow fever was present and quarantine restrictions prevented her legal exit. She informed her daughter that hundreds had already fled and carried "the seed of the disease and spread it through the country." Simpson went on to write that "in 1853 when it was so fearful in N.O. dying 300 a day the panic was not so great as is now, the Dr's from the first advise every body to leave that can. . . . Sometimes I think I will pick up and go to Marietta, Ga. There are a dozen families ready to fly."[4] Simpson's desire to flee Pensacola is typical of citizens' panic throughout the epidemic region. Fear of the contagion spurred many to disregard quarantine efforts and spread the disease as they tried to find fever-free locales. Even when communities established quarantine restrictions, uniform standards of enforcement seldom existed. Each locale acted independently.

Prior to the 1878 epidemic, because no central health agency existed, Mississippians had relied on local quarantine regulations to isolate communities from a yellow fever outbreak. Throughout the eighteenth century, many physicians believed that yellow fever outbreaks were localized in specific geographic boundaries. People would flee from infected areas or establish and maintain lines of defense around an area beset with the disease in an attempt to control the outbreak. For example, one Virginia doctor prescribed that his patients evacuate regions plagued with yellow fever.[5] As early as 1839, a prominent Texas physician reiterated the accepted contemporary belief that yellow fever could "be easily avoided by the prudent" who did not trespass into "its narrow and well defined limits."[6] At the time of the 1853 epidemic, many officials believed that yellow fever arose from specific local causes such as putrid air or general filthy living conditions, despite the fact that the 1853 epidemic struck areas once considered fever-free with equal virulence. Quarantine efforts persisted as these fever-infected locales experienced mandatory isolation from neighboring communities. Once yellow fever appeared in a locale, surrounding towns closed railroad lines and other byways in and out of the infected area. Residents secured their communities against yellow fever by isolating themselves from other regions reporting yellow fever. Particularly important were transportation lines such as the railroads.

Maintenance of quarantines in Mississippi was probably easier in 1853 than in 1878. This can be explained partly in terms of the availability of transport. Only three main railroad lines existed in the state in 1853. One main artery ran from McComb in the southwest toward Jackson, the capital. This line split just north of Grenada, with one line continuing northwest to Memphis while the other ran in a more northeasterly direction through Holly Springs, ultimately crossing into Tennessee. Closer to the Alabama border, another line operated from Meridian in the east to Corinth in the north, with stations in West Point, Macon, and Okolona. Finally, the only east-west line in 1853 bisected the state and the two other north-south lines as it crossed from Meridian through Jackson, terminating at Vicksburg on the Mississippi River.[7] These three railroad lines had only 862 miles of track in operation by 1860. Because of considerable damage to the rails during the Civil War and subsequent rebuilding problems, this figure had risen only to 990 miles by 1870.

In the 1870s, state legislation tried to encourage railroad speculation in the state, and Mississippians witnessed a limited expansion of lines. Laws such as the Subsidy Act offered a subvention of four thousand dollars per mile, and the Abatement Act allowed landowners a tax reprieve that facilitated railroad construction. Thanks also to an ample labor supply from the convict lease system that began in 1876, 1,127 railroad miles crisscrossed Mississippi by 1880. Railroads began to play a dominant role in Mississippi's expanding economy, as Vicksburg and Meridian, two key railroad cities, experienced significant population growth from 1860 to 1890.[8] The state's industrial expansion into the Progressive Era largely depended upon its ever-increasing railroad mileage.

In 1878, Mississippians took advantage of the improved railroad network to flee from yellow fever. Local officials in plague-ridden locales had difficulty establishing quarantines on expanded lines. No uniformity existed in 1878 regarding quarantine regulations along the railroads linking Mississippians; therefore, citizens could take advantage of this transportation mode as they fled from the disease and inadvertently spread the contagion.[9]

Quarantines in 1878 Mississippi, therefore, were site-specific. Two reasons account for this. First, whether or not to quarantine was a local, not a state, decision, just as in 1853—although increased railroad traffic often made a mockery of local decision making. For example, officials in Ocean Springs vigorously maintained a quarantine against any watercraft or railcars entering its environs. Those in Meridian established only a stringent surveillance of roads in their quarantine efforts. Holly Springs officials initially instituted no quarantine restrictions whatsoever, whereas Natchez enforced severe quarantines, both on land and water. Efforts to quarantine therefore varied greatly from town to town. Second, officials in charge of establishing and maintaining quarantine lines were volunteers, loosely working together to protect their towns. The Mississippi State Board of Health, created in 1877, recommended the creation of quarantines but provided no further guidance. Therefore, volunteer organizations of townspeople took matters into their own hands, sometimes using threatening displays of firepower to enforce their quarantine lines, at other times doing nothing.

Refugees fleeing yellow fever in 1878 often encountered quarantines enforced by citizens armed with double-barreled shotguns. These "shotgun quarantines" were commonplace during the epidemic months. For example, on October 20, C. L. Henderson, a railroad worker in Red Lick, wrote to a friend in Grenada that he knew "little of what was going on in the world" because of the shotgun quarantine against himself and other men who were laying track and building bridges on a ten-mile stretch of line in the region. The railroad work was completed, and he was eager to return home to Louisville, but "guards have been doubled to keep me from getting away for fear I shall scatter the fever." Neighboring locales were determined to keep the railroad workers confined in order to prevent yellow fever contagion from spreading. However, the writer stated that "When the fever gets in my camp I intend to arm the men and capture the guards and go out. I shall respect their laws only so long as I am in no danger."[10] Henderson's attitude regarding local quarantine laws expresses frustrations about shotgun quarantines but more importantly exemplifies the nonchalant attitude of many who chose to disregard quarantine regulations, regardless of armed guards, because no state laws existed to outline or enforce the quarantine regulations. On the other hand, some cities, such as Holly Springs, established no quarantine regulations at the beginning of the epidemic, believing that since it had been fever-free in the past, it was safe from the disease. Meridian quarantined pedestrian refugees but not railroad travelers; subsequently, this community experienced an outbreak of yellow fever.

In 1878, yellow fever seems to have come to Mississippi from New Orleans, at least according to the president of the Louisiana State Board of Health at the time. However, the exact origin of yellow fever's presence in New Orleans will never be known. Tracking the point of origination would be as difficult as finding the city's first host mosquito during the 1878 fever season. Yellow fever could have invaded that city from any number of sources. One possible source was the numerous trade and passenger ships that arrived at the Mississippi River Quarantine Station seventy-two miles south of New Orleans at the entrance of the waterway. The Louisiana State Board of Health created this facility in 1855, attempting to control yellow fever-infested ships on the Mississippi River in the wake of the 1853 yellow fever epidemic. Between January and April of 1878, 504 vessels cleared this quarantine station, many of them sailing from South America and the Caribbean. Freight ships continuously plied the waters between Cuba and New Orleans. During these same months, news reached the United States that yellow fever had broken out in those areas. The *Jackson Daily Clarion* announced that on March 5, 1878, "advices from Rio Janeiro [*sic*] reports that yellow fever prevails there in the city. There has been from forty to forty-five cases during the first two weeks of February."[11] Yellow fever also surfaced in Havana during this time. Despite these reports, in April the inspectors at the quarantine station allowed all vessels carrying fruit to proceed to New Orleans. Additionally, many Cuban refugees entered New Orleans during these months, because Cuba's Ten Years' War (1868–78) for independence from Spain had ended and the defeated revolutionaries sought asylum in the United States. Either of these sources could have introduced the yellow fever virus into New Orleans.[12]

Detailed information on the first outbreak of the disease in New Orleans helps to illuminate attitudes throughout the South. While the exact origin of the 1878 yellow fever epidemic remains unknown, Louisiana health officials later insisted that the source of contagion was the *Emily B. Souder*, a steamer working in the Gulf between Havana and New Orleans. On board the *Souder* approximately twenty-five sailors and nine passengers bound for New Orleans worked and traveled. After the boat reached the Mississippi River Quarantine Station on May 22, the resident physician at the station inspected the *Souder*, her crew, and passengers. His examination found a crewman named John Fordyce sick, but he declared the illness to be malarial fever and quarantined Fordyce at the station infirmary. After performing fumigation and disinfecting procedures, quarantine officials allowed the ship to continue upriver to New Orleans. Unbeknownst to the inspector, however, John E. Clark, the *Souder*'s purser, and Thomas Elliott, the ship's engineer, both carried the yellow fever virus as the ship embarked for New Orleans.[13] This situation demonstrates the difficulty in spotting the disease even when there was inspection.

The crew berthed the *Souder* at the foot of Calliope Street after reaching New Orleans on May 23, and Clark and Elliott went ashore. Clark fell ill that evening, and with a local doctor's help he went to 65 Claiborne Street, the home of Elizabeth Marshall, a widowed mulatto nurse.[14] He died on May 25, two days after he bragged that he had "beaten the quarantine doctor"—a far too common boast in Mississippi, too. Clark died at 2 a.m. and was buried by 10 a.m. the same day. Officially, his cause of death was "a malarial fever," but Clark clearly died of yellow fever. The New Orleans Board of Health sent a sanitary inspector to investigate Clark's death, and he reported on June 4 that "The nature, but more especially the *ensemble* of symptoms, the short duration of the illness, the suppression of urine, the fancy for food (always a fatal sign) shortly preceding the end, death coming after cessation of all fever, the icteric tinge after death . . . do not admit of a doubt, in my mind, that Clark died of yellow fever." City officials did not announce Clark's death immediately. According to Earnest Hardenstein, a contemporary physician practicing in Mississippi, officials did not openly announce his death for approximately two months. New Orleans bureaucrats—like their counterparts throughout Mississippi—feared public panic if a yellow fever case became public knowledge.[15]

Thomas Elliott, the *Souder*'s engineer, also died of yellow fever. After he left the ship, he rented a room at the Sailors' Boarding House on the corner of Front and Girod streets. He fell ill, and a doctor treated him for three days while he remained at his lodging. Elliott's progress did not satisfy the physician during that time, however, so he transferred Elliott to a private hospital, the Hôtel Dieu, on May 29. Elliott died the next morning at 3:00. The official death certificate listed intermittent fever as the cause of death, although a postmortem revealed yellow fever. Therefore, by order of the New Orleans Board of Health, all streets in the surrounding areas were then sprinkled with water-diluted carbolic acid. The adjoining sidewalks, yards, and gutters received the same treatment, as did all neighboring privies. Nevertheless, new cases of the disease soon developed in the wharf area on Calliope Street, on nearby Claiborne and Constance streets, and among employees at the Hôtel Dieu. On July 24, approximately eight weeks after Elliott died, the *New Orleans Daily Picayune* finally announced that yellow fever existed in the city, but it followed this news with an addendum that the disease did not threaten the city, since only strangers had contracted and died from yellow fever. By July 28, however, twenty-six people had succumbed to yellow fever in New Orleans. After learning of the deaths, officials in Mobile, Alabama, quickly organized and declared a rigid nonintercourse quarantine against New Orleans on July 30. Still, for fear of public panic and the economic losses associated with a yellow fever presence, authorities in New Orleans did not officially declare an epidemic or quarantine. The Louisiana State Board of Health, however, did announce that the fever was an extremely virulent type, based on the large number of reported cases and deaths in so short a time.[16]

After hearing of New Orleans's growing cases of yellow fever, the newly created Mississippi State Board of Health began mobilization. The legislature had established the state board of health on February 1, 1877, "for the protection of life and health and to prevent the spread of disease in the State of Mississippi, and other purposes."[17] The impetus behind the creation of the state health board, however, was more complex. According to Bradley Bond, as early as 1856, "physicians equated Mississippi's physical well-being with its economic health . . . good health fostered prosperity."[18] When the Democrats regained political control of the state, economics were part and parcel of that takeover. One of the Democrats' main complaints about the Reconstruction government in Mississippi was its wastefulness and outrageous expenditures. By creating a state board of health, the Democrats could claim to be rebuilding the economy in an unintrusive fashion that cost little in taxpayer dollars. This notion rings true, as reports from physicians later listed losses in their towns not only in terms of human lives but also in terms of monies expended for health care, funerals, and medicine, as well as unearned wages.[19]

In its regular 1878 session, however, the Mississippi legislature had amended six of the original sections of the law into twenty-one dictates, including penalties for violators. The legislature had also empowered the new board to inquire into causative factors of disease, to investigate mortalities, and to suggest preventive measures. In order to accomplish this agenda, the Mississippi State Board of Health had directed each board of supervisors in the state, "within sixty days after the passage of this law," to elect a county board of health composed of five members representing each of the five supervisors' districts. At least three of the five county board members had to be physicians, and only a doctor could serve as the chief health officer and president of the county board. County boards of health answered and reported to their board of supervisors and gave accounts to the state board of health. Therefore, at least in theory, a clear line of authority existed across the seventy-five counties in Mississippi for the dissemination of information and the gathering of health statistics. Wirt Johnston, as secretary, was the only member of the state board of health to receive compensation, an annual salary of $250. No other member or health officer in the state received any recompense for his services to the board. The act further established a $1,000 fund for health officials' travel expenses when they attended board of health meetings. The only other financial support was provision of needed forms to collect the state's demographic information and stationery for the secretary—an amount not to exceed $250. The legislative session ended on March 5, 1878, and legislators had stipulated that supervisors organize county boards of health within sixty days. But when the Mississippi State Board of Health addressed the July yellow fever outbreak in Louisiana, many of the county boards were either new or not yet organized, leaving health care in some regions at risk. Moreover, neither the county boards nor the state board was adequately funded. Therefore, both levels of health oversight were able to act only in an advisory and fact-finding capacity.[20] Nevertheless, officials such as Secretary Johnston would continuously recommend to the state and county boards of health preventives for yellow fever as the 1878 yellow fever epidemic began to spread.

When Mississippi officials initially heard rumors of the presence of yellow fever in New Orleans, they began efforts to check the spread of the disease into their state. On May 29, Wirt Johnston mailed copies of health rules and quarantine regulations to local health authorities in cities, villages, towns, or counties. These directives contained recommended quarantine and disinfectant information endorsed by the state health board. Johnston sent these guidelines as a precautionary warning, since the yellow fever season was beginning and the New Orleans rumors were numerous. He followed up with letters to the mayors of Osyka, Summit, Fort Adams, Rodney, Natchez, and Magnolia on July 30. Three of these towns—Osyka, Summit, and Magnolia—were located on a main railroad line in the southwestern portion of the state around McComb, close to the Mississippi/Louisiana border. The other cities—Fort Adams, Rodney, and Natchez—were situated on or near the Mississippi River, also in the southwestern corner of the state. Johnston was concerned about pedestrian and commercial traffic through these communities. He explained to the mayors of those cities that as of July 29, New Orleans officials had reported thirty-three yellow fever deaths, and he urged each mayor to organize a city board of health and to establish a quarantine around his respective city limits. Each mayor was to appoint men to help in the cities' efforts to safeguard themselves.[21] Johnston emphasized that Mississippi law provided blueprints for creating local boards of health for their cities under the auspices of the Mississippi State Board of Health.[22] Evidence reveals that the citizens of Osyka created a local board of health in response to Johnston's recommendation, while the other communities relied upon volunteers to cope with the upcoming disaster.[23]

On July 31, Johnston sent similar letters to other mayors throughout Mississippi. The presidents of the board of supervisors in Jackson and Harrison counties also received this correspondence. Johnston cautioned all of these officials to act swiftly: "In view of the sickly season and the prevalence of yellow fever in New Orleans, would it not be well for you to organize a Board of Health, and adopt such measures as would protect your town and improve its sanitary condition?" Eventually, all points in Mississippi received the same recommendation from Johnston.[24]

Unfortunately, the phrasing of Johnston's letter reveals the impotence of the state board of health, with Johnston attempting to persuade rather than ordering action. The board acted primarily as a collection agency for statistics regarding births, marriages, deaths, and disease investigations, especially illnesses considered to be potential epidemic threats. As a recently formed agency untested by a major epidemic, its resources and manpower would be strained to the limit by the 1878 yellow fever epidemic. There was no money for quarantine costs or disinfectant purchases for communities in time of need. Mississippi lawmakers simply outlined the duties of the state board to include ensuring cooperation of quarantine commissioners and sanitary authorities during any threatened danger, reporting vital statistics and information on sanitary conditions to the governor, and outlining other duties that the circuit clerks would fulfill regarding the compilation of vital statistics for the board. The law also stipulated that if a county board of health, created under the auspices of this act, ascertained that "any matter in their county calculated in their opinion, to produce or to aggravate or cause the spread of any epidemic, endemic or contagious disease, or to cause typhoid fever or other disease, or in any way injuriously affect public health, the board of supervisors of each county may declare the same a nuisance." The judge of the circuit court in the district where the "nuisance" existed could then try the responsible party within five days. The district attorney acted on behalf of the board as its prosecutor. If any person violated the regulations of a county board of health, the district attorney could request a fine for each offense, "in any sum not exceeding fifty dollars, or by imprisonment in the county jail not exceeding one month, or by both such fine and imprisonment."[25]

All of these measures might have helped if local boards had been in place. However, the 1878 yellow fever epidemic soon became too extensive for local authorities and the state board of health to manage with such limited resources. With unfunded mandates from the Mississippi legislature and inadequate personnel in the state board of health, the state was woefully unprepared.

The probable source of contagion for Mississippi was a ship that traveled the trade routes on the Mississippi and Ohio rivers. On July 19 the towboat *John Porter* left New Orleans on a run to the Ohio River. It stopped in Vicksburg on July 25 to bury two crew members, an engineer and a fireman. Sextons buried these men in the Vicksburg City Cemetery. According to the *Memphis Daily Appeal,* the *Porter* was "a floating charnel-house carrying death and destruction to nearly all who had anything to do with her. Twenty-three persons died on her from the time she left New Orleans until she anchored near Pittsburgh."[26]

Despite the reported deaths of the *Porter,* Paul Stoltz of Vicksburg signed on as a crew member to replace the dead fireman. He continued on the boat until July 29, when it reached Cairo, Illinois. At that point, Stoltz began to exhibit mild symptoms of illness. Back in Vicksburg, the *Herald* had published on July 26 an editorial urging a strict quarantine against New Orleans traffic and mail. Vicksburg officials, however, did not immediately respond to the *Herald's* alarm, because towns hesitated to initiate quarantines so as not to interrupt commerce; therefore, when illness forced Stoltz to return to Vicksburg, he was able to do so unhindered.[27]

Stoltz arrived in Vicksburg on August 7. Not feeling well, he stopped at a drugstore where locals asked him about the yellow fever deaths on board the *Porter.* He replied, "Why, they no more had it than I have now." However, because of Stoltz's unhealthy appearance and most probably his recent tour on the *Porter,* the Vicksburg health authorities intervened and hospitalized him that same day. Stoltz died two days later of yellow fever. The city's health officials then announced the infiltration of the dreaded disease on August 10.[28] After the announcement, some people exhibited alarm. William H. Hardy, the entrepreneur and eventual founder of Hattiesburg, wrote to his wife, Hattie Lott Hardy, in Mobile to warn her of the impending spread of yellow fever. He instructed her to join him in Meridian and not to let his mother remain in Mobile, as "yellow fever is spreading in N. O. and will be in Mobile soon."[29]

Some towns along the Mississippi Gulf Coast had already established a quarantine against New Orleans after news of the yellow scourge reached those areas in July. Health officials who attempted to maintain quarantine restrictions, however, often found themselves at odds with local business interests, particularly along the Gulf Coast, which enjoyed a lucrative economy as a tourist destination. Often, towns in basically the same location differed as to quarantine regulations and enforcement. Towns had to work independently of each other in a most stressful situation with no clear guidance and little authority. The *Pascagoula Democrat-Star* reported on July 26 that Pascagoula and Mississippi City "do not believe there is any probability of fever getting into our ports this summer, as a strict quarantine is kept up at all the towns." These restrictions were to be enforced even if "it does displease some."[30] Not all the coastal cities reacted as these two communities did, however. Biloxi had a less stringent quarantine, since its health officials did not want to fight local interests and possibly stymie its economy. Handsboro officials also did not establish strong quarantine restrictions during late July and August because of that city's role as a vacation spot and as a haven for New Orleans refugees. Hotels in these two locales were full as

New Orleanians fled the yellow fever and others simply enjoyed the coastal hospitality. Business was brisk; quarantine restrictions would hinder if not halt those economic opportunities. Quarantines consequently proved to be a difficult logistical hurdle for Mississippians to jump during the 1878 yellow fever epidemic.[31]

One Mississippi city that appears to have had a successful quarantine during September 1878 was the state capital, Jackson, presumably the place with the most effective governmental organization to maintain a strict quarantine. Whether it was thanks to quarantines or not, Jackson recorded only two yellow fever deaths in September. Although few deaths occurred in Jackson that month, increased quarantine security greatly disrupted charitable efforts and life for the city's residents during the epidemic. One example of the difficulties behind quarantine lines involved the Griffith and Griffing families, two prominent Mississippi families. Benjamin Whitfield Griffith was a banker in Jackson and a graduate of Mississippi College. Cora Griffing was from Forest Grove Plantation near Pattison and was a graduate of the Female Seminary in Port Gibson. The two had met in 1877 at the Cooper's Well resort, a destination famous for its mineral waters and baths.[32] When Griffith and Griffing met, they developed a great affection for one another and decided to marry. The wedding was set for September 1878. However, the epidemic that fall prevented their marriage. Moreover, they were unable even to communicate with one another because of Jackson's quarantine restrictions, so it was impossible to make wedding plans at that time.[33]

Griffith also had another problem exacerbated by the quarantine restrictions in the Jackson vicinity during September. His family farm was about a mile north of Jackson. When news of Vicksburg's infestation with yellow fever reached Jackson, his family and several others with their servants moved to the Griffith place to wait out the pestilence and quarantine. As the weeks passed, Griffith became agitated about the safety of a cousin of his from Clinton, a town between Jackson and Vicksburg. Correspondence with his cousin was impossible because of mail quarantines in the region, so Griffith asked his African-American handyman, John L. Dennis, to deliver a message. Dennis would have to travel through quarantine zones to accomplish the task.[34]

Griffith made all the arrangements for Dennis to carry the message. Mounting a little gray pony, the handyman headed off to Clinton to deliver Griffith's letter. He also carried a "pas [sic]" (certificate of health) with him so that he could travel through the quarantine lines. He later recounted that he worked his "way around quarantines to the out skirts of Clinton where there was a shot gun guarentine [sic] station." The guards "started to waving and hollering at me when I was quite a distance frome [sic] them." Cautiously approaching the armed men, he raised his hands to show that he had a letter in one and a pass in the other.

The guards then ordered him to throw the letters down and retreat. The armed men approached the letters and, after examining them, took Griffith's correspondence to Clinton. Dennis waited the better part of the day for a reply. When the guard finally returned with an answer, he laid the letter on the ground and rode away. Only then could Dennis pick up the reply and be on his way. After he returned to the Griffith place, the family warmly greeted Dennis.[35]

Along the Mississippi Gulf Coast, the month of September was also pivotal regarding quarantine regulations and charitable donations. Quarantines were uppermost in the minds of the coast's citizens. George Nicholson, a local health official in Hancock County, commented on September 5 that Hancock County had established a quarantine station: "the Board of Health this morning established a Quarantine Station at Brown's Island, five miles below Pearlington. Vessels from infected ports will be detained six days." Pearlington was a small post village located eight miles from the mouth of the Pearl River that divides Mississippi from Louisiana. However, Nicholson indicated that Bay St. Louis had not established a quarantine at this time, nor had "intermediate places." By September 12, Pearlington officials had also enacted a mail quarantine; under the requirements of this health measure, second- and third-class mail entering the city had to be fumigated. Officials there must have believed that first-class mail was exempt from contagion and appear to have accepted the fomite theory of how yellow fever spread, the belief that yellow fever contagion could adhere to concrete objects. Yet, Dr. J. A. Mead, the health officer in Pearlington, expressed his desire for quarantines when he stated in the *Pascagoula Democrat-Star:* "This unwelcome visitor [yellow fever] is gradually and truly visiting many a rustic home that never dreamed of it, and leaves a vacant chair and ofttimes more than one in every household where it enters."[36] Certainly there were doubts about the effectiveness of the quarantines, in spite of Mead's observation. They were inconvenient, and they were not keeping yellow fever contagion at bay.

Because of the lack of government officials in many Mississippi towns and crossroads, local doctors across the state assumed greater responsibilities as a result of yellow fever's ever-broadening presence. The state board of health should have been coordinating relief efforts, but instead, local doctors were taking on a more independent role. They were forced to make critical decisions, often with no clear mandates from the state board. This dilemma was evident along the Gulf Coast as well as other points in Mississippi. For example, during the epidemic, Dr. Charles Pelaez was the quarantine physician and health officer for Harrison County, midway between New Orleans and Mobile. The New Orleans and Mobile Railroad ran in an east-west direction through the county, with stops at numerous towns and villages along the route. Pelaez reported that Harrison County quarantined early against the cities of New Orleans and Mobile, "but owing to our utter inability to make it effectual . . . we were compelled to allow our ports to remain open; fugitives from the infected city [New Orleans] [were] pouring in our midst, both by land and water." Therefore, Pelaez was able to trace the first cases of yellow fever in Harrison County cities to infected refugees from New Orleans. When news of local fever cases reached Pelaez, he usually instructed the city to disinfect everything with carbolic acid or sulphate of iron. He did not believe that disinfectants stopped yellow fever, but perhaps the public was psychologically appeased by these recommendations. He also advised public officials to boil bedding and clothes that had been used by yellow fever patients and to burn all their soiled mattresses. Pelaez stated in his official report, however, that these control efforts were "in error. In my humble opinion the only agent that will effectually destroy yellow fever is an intense degree of cold." He ended his observations by stating that "panic stricken" refugees from New Orleans had sought safety along the coast and "spread the disease nearly over the whole county."[37]

The failure of quarantine measures in Harrison County illustrates the conflict between business interests and health officials. Those involved in the tourist business believed the quarantine to be misguided in the first place. Tourist destinations in Harrison County, particularly for New Orleanians, included such cities as Biloxi, Mississippi City, and Handsboro. Refugees from New Orleans gathered at the numerous hotels and boardinghouses in these locations. Business was too good to enforce a quarantine strictly, adding frustration to an already stressed populace.

Quarantine regulations hindered everyday activities during the 1878 epidemic. For example, fear of yellow fever contagion and shotgun quarantines caused educational institutions to postpone September opening dates. The Mississippi Military Institute in Pass Christian announced that its next session would begin on the first Monday in November instead of its usual September opening. In Jackson County, officials canceled the school session in Scranton until November 1. Further inland, Meridian Female College delayed its opening until October 1, and local newspapers announced that "Oxford University [the University of Mississippi] will open on the 31st of October. This postponement has been made on account of the epidemic prevailing throughout the land." The epidemic proved to be more virulent than first anticipated by the University of Mississippi's board of trustees; as a result, the school session was again delayed until November 21. Because of this lengthy postponement, the trustees in 1878 canceled all Christmas holidays except December 25. The board even suggested that in order for faculty members to complete their academic courses, instructors should consider teaching on Saturdays. Mississippi College, located near Jackson and Cooper's Well, announced that it would begin its fall session on October 23 instead of September 25, but the college had to postpone opening yet again, to November 6, as yellow fever continued to wreak havoc in Mississippi. Even Sunday school teachers had to interrupt that instruction. In Handsboro, the local paper announced that "Sabbath-school" at the Masonic Hall was canceled indefinitely until the city was "again healthy."[38]

Quarantines failed again and again because, to many, the quarantine itself seemed worse than the risk of contracting the disease. The general lack of local and state authority resulted in quarantine failures. Mississippians living in towns along the Mississippi River attempted to isolate themselves from yellow fever contagion through quarantine boundaries, as did their counterparts in the state's interior. These quarantine plans were virtually impossible to maintain, however. Many Mississippians even believed that quarantine restrictions punished the populace by denying them access to necessary food and supplies. Unless forced to do so by armed guards, some of the state's citizens refused to observe quarantine regulations. One contemporary writer wrote that a quarantine is the "invention of the devil," and "there is nothing in the history of despotism [that] can surpass it."[39]

Regardless of this strongly worded complaint, three towns along the Mississippi River—Port Gibson, Vicksburg, and Greenville—tried desperately in September to enforce quarantines against yellow fever. These communities believed that their location on and near the Mississippi made them particularly vulnerable to yellow fever contagion, as historically yellow fever had spread along that waterway. Therefore, the towns' power brokers took matters into their own hands.

Port Gibson, the county seat of Claiborne County, is situated on Bayou Pierre, seven miles from the Mississippi River. Prior to the announcement of yellow fever, approximately fifteen hundred people lived in this town. After yellow fever appeared, the population dwindled to seven hundred as citizens sought safety in the countryside.[40] The first case of yellow fever in Port Gibson had been identified on August 3. The victim was August Samuelson, a mailman and railroad worker. On July 23, Samuelson had come into contact with crew members from the tugboat *John D. Porter* when it had landed at Port Gibson to unload some iron railroad ties and mail. This is the same vessel that went on to Vicksburg and docked there on July 25. The local doctor reported that George Goodrich, an African American, nursed Samuelson at Louder House, a local boarding establishment, but Samuelson died on August 8. Goodrich died a week later, also of yellow fever. After word of the deaths spread through Port Gibson, there was a mass exodus of citizens for two days. Eventually, between four and five hundred people left as fast as they could; even so, by the beginning of September, health officials reported 400 cases of fever and 55 deaths.[41]

The example of Port Gibson seems to indicate that quarantines were largely ineffective when they were imposed locally and only after the fever had already appeared. The scenario played out in Port Gibson and other towns across Mississippi consisted first of yellow fever's appearance, then the exodus of panicked populations, and finally an established quarantine with local patrols attempting to enforce it.

During September, the Claiborne County Board of Health quarantined the entire county's boundaries along the Mississippi River. The region, however, could not tend to the ever-increasing number of yellow fever cases and deaths, so nurses from the Howard Association in New Orleans received permission to enter Port Gibson on September 2, crossing quarantine lines. By the time they arrived to help, "the distress [was] very great, [and] the dying [had] no one to give them a drink of water."[42] Port Gibson's situation demonstrates the futility of quarantines and citizens' reliance upon charitable organizations. The Mississippi government offered no help, so citizens themselves filled the void and looked to outside intervention for even the most basic provisions.

As a result of the state's lack of involvement, the crisis would play out at the local level. The economic ramifications of quarantines created conflict between health officials, who advocated quarantines to protect citizens, and business owners, who relied upon commerce for their livelihood. Cities with a lucrative tourist industry realized that quarantine lines created economic hardships for the entire city economy, not just individual businesses. The tourist business enjoyed by such cities created a trickle-down effect that helped all aspects of a city's economy. Visitors brought money to boat owners, grocers, laborers, suppliers, and manufacturers of items ranging from lumber used to construct the hostelries to surrey drivers transporting visitors to and from the docks.

Other areas also wrestled with whether or not to quarantine. On August 2 the Jackson County Board of Health issued a rail and water quarantine. Editors of the *Pascagoula Democrat-Star* reflected this struggle: "Some think they [the Jackson County Board of Health] were somewhat hasty in their action, while others heartily approve their course and think they did what was wise and proper."[43] This editorial summarizes well Mississippians' experience regarding quarantines. It was a dilemma faced by local boards of health and businesses that often operated at cross-purposes. For example, in Pascagoula, a merchant reported to the newspaper that he had ordered groceries from a supplier in Mobile. The Alabama businessman informed the Mississippi grocer that he could not ship the food because Mobile had imposed a quarantine against the Gulf Coast. The newspaper editor opined that "As we have no yellow fever on the coast we see no sense in Mobile quarantining us, and thus depriving our people of something to eat."[44] It was a local decision, based on local notions of what might help. For example, at Vicksburg they fired cannon in attempts to clear foul air that they believed harbored miasma. Oddly, the measure seemed effective, since the smoke from the cannon thwarted mosquitoes' activities. Health officers also quarantined some items believed capable of transporting fomites but did not quarantine others. Until scientists discovered yellow fever's etiology, quarantines and other control efforts aimed at the disease saved few lives and were only partially effective, as no mosquito control and eradication measures existed to halt its spread.

Although the Mississippi State Board of Health exhibited concern to establish quarantines and recommend proper measurements of carbolic acid to disinfect in July and August, most people did not believe that yellow fever would reach epidemic proportions. Carbolic acid was extremely effective in killing insects; therefore, health officials stumbled upon another partially effective remedy. Annual visitations of the disease had been somewhat mild since the 1853 epidemic. In the Mississippi River region, therefore, even Stoltz's death did not greatly alarm the general disease. Many Mississippians disregarded local quarantine regulations and warnings, often even welcoming yellow fever refugees into their midst as the scourge spread throughout the state. Mississippians' attitudes toward quarantines reflected the general mind-set toward regulations. They had flaunted Reconstruction regulations—and those who were now their elected officials had encouraged them to do so. Often flagrantly ignoring quarantine measures, Mississippians traveled throughout the state seeking safety.

A good example of this disregard for quarantine restrictions and the lack of apprehension exhibited by many Mississippians involves Mary and Albert Buford, who lived near Water Valley in Yalobusha County. At the time of the epidemic, Mary was seventy years old and owned property from a previous marriage on what is today known as Lover's Lane and Gulf Hills in Ocean Springs. Hoping to resolve a dispute over the sale of a portion of her Gulf Hills property, she first traveled alone by train from Water Valley (in the northern half of the state) to Biloxi (on the Gulf Coast). After arriving in Biloxi, she boarded a boat to sail across Biloxi Bay to Ocean Springs on August 2. Mary insisted upon immediately investigating her property, even though news of yellow fever was widespread and several coastal communities, including Mississippi City and Pascagoula, had already established strict quarantine regulations regarding travel in and out of those towns. Because of its tourist business, however, Ocean Springs had not established a clear quarantine policy, and Mary was able to travel freely to that city.

Mary first received news about the growing yellow fever danger in Mississippi from her husband's dire warnings in a letter. On August 8 he wrote that he did not "like the look of things. The first thing that you know your retreat will be cut off. But I don't know enough to advise you. . . . I am getting uneasy as to how you are to get home without contracting the disease your self or bringing it home in your clothing or trunk and giv[ing] it to the rest of us." Two days later, he further demonstrated concern about her return trip home: "I think you had better . . . come home at once as the trains on our Road may stop at any time."[45]

By August 14, Mary was alarmed at the developing yellow fever situation along the Gulf Coast. Albert had already reported to her that the nearest large town, Grenada, had declared fifty yellow fever cases and four deaths. He had even predicted on August 8 that the "fever is bound to be epidemic." Mary responded emotionally to her husband, imploring, "May God stay the terrible scourge ere it reaches my precious husband. I am so torn with conflicted thoughts that I am almost crazy. If I had the means to come I might bring the fever into my own family and cause sorrow instead of joy. I am advised not to attempt to but if I had our business here so that I could leave it I think I would come unless you opposed it. I am not thinking of myself, it is of you."[46]

The heartrending exchange between Mary and Albert continued throughout the month of August and revealed growing panic and concern about yellow fever and each other. Their letters also highlight the fact that Mississippians were ignorant about the mode of yellow fever transmission, as Albert, unaware of the mosquito vector, warned Mary about bringing home yellow fever in her clothing or her luggage. Mary correctly reiterated that belief with her poignant discussion about whether she should come home and risk carrying the disease to her family or try to stay in Ocean Springs and at least keep Albert safe from her. She could have been a "carrier" and infected Water Valley—or so she thought.

Both husband and wife also reported local news in their respective towns and offered medical advice. Mary was particularly anxious because she was not with her husband during this dangerous time. On August 21 she reported a yellow fever death in Ocean Springs but stressed to her husband that "disinfectants are being used all over town," attempting to assure Albert that the situation in Ocean Springs was under control. "I will try to be patient and trust in God for a happy reunion with my dear husband again on earth," she longingly concluded. As an afterthought, she asked, "have you put camphor in your shoes? If not do it by all means," revealing her belief that the strong smell of camphor deterred yellow fever transmission. Mary continued her medicinal thoughts in her August 25 letter to Albert. She had not been feeling well, so she reassured him, "I took a quinine pill this morning, and think I will be all right in a day or two." Interestingly, she informed her husband in the same letter that "the mosquitoes are *awful*. There is no peace in the house without a smoke [fumigation method], so unpleasant, you don't know how I want to fly home." By the time Mary commu-

nicated this news to Water Valley, quarantine restrictions were being more strin-
gently enforced throughout some yellow fever areas, and Mary had no chance of
returning to her beloved husband.[47]

On August 29, Mary spoke for every Mississippian who was caught behind
quarantine lines when she wrote: "everything like business is paralyzed, and what
a long time it [yellow fever] has to run yet. I am half crazy to see you and be at
home. It does seem *too long* to wait until frost." On September 5 she sadly informed Albert that she was again not feeling well. She added, "Oh how I long to
be with you again. *It looks like I am floating away from you forever, the outlook is
so gloomy, so sad.*"[48] She was right. Albert received a telegram on September 12
informing him that his beloved Mary "Died Last night [at] nine thirty. Will be
buried at her request at this place."[49] Mary never realized her dream of being reunited with her husband.

As revealed in the Bufords' letters, August was a pivotal month in 1878 Mississippi. After its initial introduction by way of the Mississippi River in July, the
contagion spread throughout the state during August and September. Many cities
that had never experienced yellow fever in epidemic proportions were in Bronze
John's grip by the middle of August as the disease continued its ever-widening
swath into the state along the more numerous railroad lines. People fleeing to
the countryside to escape the disease inadvertently carried mosquitoes on their
clothes or in the railroad cars or transported the yellow fever virus in their systems, thus spreading the dreaded saffron scourge.

During July and August, coastal cities in Hancock, Harrison, and Jackson
counties persisted in their attempts to enforce sketchy quarantine regulations.
Refugees from New Orleans, however, continued to flood into many areas of
this coastal region, thereby spreading yellow fever. Bay St. Louis, a small resort
village on the seashore in Hancock County, was one coastal city involved in this
quarantine/refugee situation that exemplifies the typical response. Usually, the
initial response depended on local decisions. Bay St. Louis's citizens controlled
their own quarantine laws as city and health officials saw fit and not as suggested
by the Mississippi State Board of Health.

Bay St. Louis was situated on the New Orleans and Mobile Railroad line,
only fifty-two miles from New Orleans. In late July the estimated population of
three thousand in the small city had approximately doubled as New Orleanians
fled their homes. Those New Orleanians who had the financial means and who
believed they were not acclimated to the disease fled the city. Bay St. Louis was
one of the closest havens along the Gulf Coast and a community that had not initially quarantined against New Orleans. This year, however, the refuge that New
Orleanians sought was not to be found.[50]

On July 28, doctors diagnosed M. Ballentine, a native of the Bay St. Louis area, with yellow fever. That same date, twenty-six people died of Yellow Jack in New Orleans. Ballentine's, however, was the first known coastal case of yellow fever. Health officials stated that he was "well cared for and recovered." By August 14, Rebecca Necaise had contracted the disease, and she died shortly thereafter. The contagion spread rapidly throughout the Bay St. Louis area and surrounding Piney Woods. Local health officials *then* recognized yellow fever on the Mississippi coast, and Mississippi towns along the coast immediately quarantined against New Orleans. Mobile, also fearing yellow fever, had issued a quarantine against New Orleans on July 27. Once again these efforts were futile, because the yellow fever virus was already in their locales.[51] Moreover, quarantines were only effective when citizens complied with them and communities had enough officials and volunteers to enforce them rigidly.

Officials of Jackson County appeared to be more concerned with quarantines than those of Harrison or Hancock County. Jackson County was not as involved in the New Orleans tourist trade, as it was further from Louisiana and did not have a large expanse of beachfront property. On July 29, the board of health in Scranton (present-day Pascagoula) convened for the purpose of organizing against the potential invasion of yellow fever. Scranton was approximately thirty-six miles from Mobile. In the previous week's edition of the *Pascagoula Democrat-Star,* reports had warned this coastal city and its environs about the growing yellow fever threat in New Orleans, so Scranton's health officials were eager to begin preparations to thwart the spread of the disease into their city. This board decided that a committee of three would investigate the cost of enacting and maintaining a quarantine. The committee also purchased some beacons, which were to be erected at the quarantine's boundary lines to alert those attempting to cross into their community that they were violating a quarantine. The devices cost three dollars. Some of the city's citizens believed that the members of the board of health were acting hastily, while others approved. Still others clung to the hope that the disease might not reach epidemic proportions. The local paper editorialized hopefully: "The yellow fever has not yet been declared an epidemic in New Orleans, and it may not assume that form this season." Nevertheless, the city's board of health was not going to take any chances.[52]

Scranton officials clearly outlined quarantine limitations for the trains and ships coming into their city. They explained that those who ignored the restrictions would be fined. Scranton officials enacting the quarantine were prominent men in the community socially and economically and were therefore representative of the power elite. For example, the families of E. F. Griffin and S. A. McInnis, two of the six officials involved in the decision, were founders of Jackson County, and Griffin, a Democrat, had been elected to the state legislature in 1877.[53] Their insistence regarding the quarantines was consequently accepted as the correct procedure for the city. Scranton's health officers also adopted a resolution that stated: "the city of New Orleans is hereby declared an infected port until further notice, and no railroad train, car or engine shall, after the 29th day of July, stop within the limits of Jackson County when coming from said city." This resolution further stipulated that if a train did come from New Orleans, "it shall be allowed to travel at a rate of speed not less than ten miles an hour when delivering mails." Sailing vessels arriving from New Orleans had to wait at the mouth of the Pascagoula River until the quarantine physician was able to inspect the ship. Health officials also empowered bridge tenders to close their bridges to all vessels not flying an all-clear flag from the quarantine station. Additionally, no person "who has been in the city of New Orleans within the last ten days pending their arrival in said county" was allowed into Jackson County. Dr. Blount, the quarantine physician and a member of the original quarantine investigative committee, appointed Dr. John J. Harry to oversee matters in Ocean Springs as well as in Jackson County. Furthermore, a suitable person (described in the local paper as a member of "the true democracy hereabout") was to be chosen at each community to enforce this resolution and "to arrest and prosecute any violations thereof."[54] Such a statement suggests the odd mix of state and local politics involved. The Mississippi power elite had claimed a return to democracy with the election of the Democrats, but Democrats advocated that power should be vested "hereabouts" rather than statewide. A notification of the quarantine resolution appeared in the *Pascagoula Democrat-Star* and served as a public warning. Jackson County's officials also alerted the superintendent of the New Orleans and Mobile Railroad to the county's actions. The paper further expressed the feelings of most citizens when it stated that Mississippians along the coast now had "quarantine to the right of us, quarantine to the left of us," referring to the Gulf Coast's position between Mobile and New Orleans and impending commercial interruption.[55] Despite these multiple quarantine efforts, yellow fever appeared in the coastal communities.

Local health officials exercised their authority to establish quarantine stations under an act created by the state legislature on March 24, 1876. This law allowed for the establishment of quarantines from May 1 through November 15 during yellow fever years. The quarantine could last for a longer period if officials deemed it necessary "to prevent the introduction of contagious, infectious and other diseases among the citizens." By this same act, the quarantine station was to fly a yellow flag if Bronze John was detected upon any of the ships being investigated. The inspectors assessed each ship searched a fee of five dollars. During the 1878 epidemic, city officials collected many fees as shipping traffic went to and from Jackson County, a region whose economic welfare rested on maritime commerce.[56]

Gulf Coast quarantines often led to massive confusion for travelers caught in their web. Another good example of problems that arose because of no uniform directives from the state board of health occurred on the steamer *Pearl River,* which carried passengers and freight between New Orleans and the Mississippi Gulf Coast. It left New Orleans on July 31 for a pleasure cruise to Mississippi even as the yellow fever epidemic began to spread. After a "lovely" trip to Biloxi, the quarantine officer in Ocean Springs ordered off the boat thirty-one passengers and some of its cargo, even though the vessel had just passed Bay St. Louis, Pass Christian, Handsboro, Mississippi City, Beauvoir, and Biloxi without being stopped for inspection. Captain Poitevent, in command of the *Pearl River,* then received a letter of permission from Dr. Harry, the appointed physician at the Ocean Springs Quarantine Station, to proceed to Moss Point, a small town located on the Pascagoula River next to Scranton. Officials at the quarantine station had fumigated the contents of the steamer and disinfected the passengers properly to adhere to Jackson County's health standards.[57] When the boat arrived in Scranton, another quarantine officer then ordered the *Pearl River,* its freight, crew, and nine passengers into quarantine. The local board of health had empowered the local doctor as the quarantine physician, and apparently with their political support, his position was strong enough that he could enforce the local quarantine restrictions. Captain Poitevent obeyed Blount's orders and moved the ship to the quarantine station outside the port of Scranton. After completing quarantine requirements at Scranton, the *Pearl River* quickly sought refuge in Harrison County's Bay of Biloxi, which had not established a quarantine.[58] This incident highlights the vagaries of the quarantine situation along the Mississippi Gulf Coast. This erratic establishment and maintenance of quarantine lines continued throughout Mississippi.

Economic considerations often overrode quarantine recommendations from local health officials, as in the case of the *Pearl River.* Because of their dependence upon commerce and tourist dollars, cities along the Mississippi Gulf Coast did not stop the ship. Harrison and Hancock counties, therefore, did not enforce a quarantine. Commercial dependence on New Orleans's trade via the railroad and maritime routes led the majority of the coastal cities to avoid establishing quarantines in July or August. Collectively, the string of cities or "watering places" along the Mississippi Gulf Coast—Bay St. Louis, Pass Christian, Mississippi City, Biloxi, Ocean Springs, and Scranton (East and West Pascagoula)—was known as the "Six Sisters." These communities offered a safe refuge and summer pleasures such as fishing, sunbathing, and various other entertainments to New Orleanians who wished to escape the heat of the city or in times of yellow fever outbreaks. Handsboro was also an important commercial-industrial village in this area. Three of these cities—Biloxi, Handsboro, and Pass Christian—

expressed concerns over any quarantine restrictions. These cities in Harrison County were close to New Orleans and consequently had more commercial connections through the tourist trade to that city. One reporter expressed those communities' concerns when he urged: "It seems to be the unanimous opinion of our citizens that to declare a quarantine against New Orleans is both unnecessary and inexpedient. We earnestly hope that the board of health of Harrison county will look at the matter in the same light, for the small amount of fever in New Orleans does not justify any reasonable man in raising such a hue and cry for a quarantine."[59]

Famous for their hotels and salubrious atmospheres, the "Six Sisters" aggressively advertised their attractions in New Orleans and local papers throughout the summer. As early as August 2, reports affirmed that Biloxi was "overflowing with strangers" and that the hotels and boardinghouses "are reaping a rich harvest." "No place on the coast is better patronized this summer than this place," boasted the *Pascagoula Democrat-Star*.[60] Mississippi City also welcomed daily guests to the Barnes and Tegarden hotels as tourists disembarked from the train that ran through Harrison County from New Orleans. These two resorts on the Gulf of Mexico are just two examples of the many establishments that were available and that advertised weekly for more visitors. Naturally, hotel and boardinghouse owners did not want quarantine restrictions hindering their businesses and restricting the flow of customers. Additionally, the flow of food items and dry goods necessary to maintain the establishments would be greatly reduced by quarantine regulations.[61]

In Biloxi, the oystermen were vexed with other towns' quarantine restrictions, because the "oyster trade will not open . . . before late October." Quarantine restrictions on the railroad and maritime routes prevented the bivalves from being shipped out of Biloxi to main distribution points. Many citizens in Ocean Springs also disagreed with enforcing quarantine regulations, despite the efforts of the quarantine station. They protested "so loud and deep . . . that last Monday the board of health visited that place to hold a consultation with her citizens and see for themselves the exact condition of things." At the meeting, residents told health officials that the quarantine injured "business interests" and that they wanted "free intercourse with New Orleans."[62] It was all very democratic, as well as Democratic, emphasizing local decision making and vesting power in local economic interests.

Refugees often created further problems for local citizenry as they sought safety in regions perceived to be healthy, thus taxing already overburdened resources. Officials in Stonewall, a small settlement north of the Bay of Biloxi in Harrison County, reported that there was much activity in their area because of refugees and that food supplies were dwindling as a result. Stonewall's residents, nevertheless, were against a quarantine, because it "would keep out grub, and then we would certainly starve. Give us grub and no quarantine."[63]

People fleeing yellow fever usually encountered several different quarantine scenarios. Quarantine regulations sometimes prohibited the entry of strangers into a town, while other locations welcomed refugees because of false assumptions, such as the idea that being free of yellow fever in previous years indicated that the community as a whole was immune. If an area had not previously been visited by yellow fever, that town incorrectly assumed that it could not be affected during this particular outbreak, rather like the recent situation on the Mississippi Gulf Coast when people refused to leave their homes during Hurricane Katrina because they had been unaffected by Hurricane Camille. Holly Springs was one such town whose citizens believed yellow fever was unlikely during August 1878.

Holly Springs had apparently never experienced severe outbreaks of yellow fever. This city is in the northern portion of the state, situated on an elevated ridge; it is a relatively isolated locale, even though the town is located on the Mississippi Central Railroad line. This particular section of railroad track was completed prior to 1861 but had sustained considerable damage between 1861 and 1865.[64] However, by 1878 the Mississippi Central was operational and refugees packed into its cars. That year the population of Holly Springs was approximately four thousand, and the town enjoyed a reputation as a healthy locale, "remarkable for the purity of its atmosphere, salubrity of climate, and general healthfulness in every respect."[65] Most contemporaries believed that yellow fever could not exist in high, dry altitudes; therefore, citizens in Holly Springs believed themselves to be safe.[66]

Since Holly Springs had never officially recorded a case of yellow fever prior to the 1878 epidemic, the city was lulled into a false sense of security. In early August, officials moved U.S. troops garrisoned at New Orleans to Holly Springs. However, a case of yellow fever among the soldiers stationed in the city appeared as early as August 12.[67] The soldier had probably arrived in the city already sick with yellow fever. Perhaps the town leaders chose to ignore this warning sign in an effort to perpetuate Holly Springs's reputation as a fever-free location or to avoid any disturbance in commerce that would result from a quarantine. Whatever the reason, when news of yellow fever in Grenada and Memphis reached Holly Springs, its leaders and citizens openly invited refugees from these locations, especially Grenada, into their midst. The *New Orleans Times* described the "Noble Hearted Little City" that welcomed refugees fleeing yellow fever: "The report that yellow fever has broken out amongst the United States troops garrisoning this place is utterly without foundation. The town is clean and healthy and there is no symptom of the outbreak . . . in fact, we have declared against quarantine, and have thrown open our hospitality to all our sister cities. . . . We apprehend nothing like even a brush with yellow jack, much less an epidemic."[68]

Holly Springs's health officials and citizenry underestimated the virulence of yellow fever in 1878. Believing that their city was safe because of its elevation, they did not implement quarantines. Since no state laws forced communities to establish quarantines, the decision-making elites were free to do as they wished. The city's officials and citizens opened "their hearts, houses, and purses" to those fleeing the yellow fever plague. The result was deadly, with a first yellow fever death recorded on August 26. Many Holly Springs residents, however, continued to believe that the disease was confined to other locales. One citizen of the town, a man named McCroskey, explained in late August that six cases of yellow fever existed in Holly Springs, but he noted that five of them were from Grenada and one was from Memphis. "These are all Reffugees [sic]," affirmed McCroskey, who continued by warning that "the News from all points where the yellow fever is Epidemic is Terable [sic] on the increase. . . . We hope it will not spread in this place."[69]

Unfortunately, by August 31 three more adults had died of yellow fever in Holly Springs, as well as three children, all lifelong residents of the city. The three children were the daughters of George Buchanan and Victoria Nunnally Buchanan. Buchanan had been a Confederate soldier from Kentucky who had gone to Holly Springs to convalesce after the battle at Corinth in 1862; he remained to marry his nurse, Victoria Nunnally. By 1872 the couple had three daughters, Susan Dean, Nancy Warren, and Fannie Dean. In August 1878, however, Buchanan and his wife had to endure the heartbreak of watching all three of their daughters die of yellow fever within a ten-day period. This type of tragedy occurred repeatedly throughout Mississippi during this time. Holly Springs was no longer able to brag about its healthy environment. By the end of August the population of the city had dwindled to approximately fifteen hundred because most of its citizens had become refugees themselves. By September 1 Dr. J. P. Dromgoole reported that "the disease had become general and rages with fury, and telegrams poured over the land telling that the city of flowers had become the city of death."[70] Yellow fever continued to extend its grip across Mississippi.

Quarantine regulations lacked uniformity throughout the epidemic. Nevertheless, they affected all aspects of life, including political activity. For example, cities in Leflore County reported a marked decrease in their national congressional election turnouts for the November 5 election. Greenwood is the largest city in this Delta county and the county seat. The *Yazoo Valley Flag* explained that far fewer votes were cast in the congressional election in 1878 than in 1877. Table 1 illustrates the effects of the epidemic on the congressional election turnout in that county. The *Yazoo Valley Flag* explained the sharp decrease in total

Table 1. Leflore County congressional elections turnout, 1877 and 1878

Locales	1877	1878
Minter City	381	38
Shell Mound	484	39
Greenwood	587	53
Roebuck	271	23
Rising Sun	93	0
Sheppardstown	255	17
Sidon	101	11
Total	2172	191

Source: *Yazoo Valley Flag,* November 22, 1878.

votes cast as follows: "In this, as in many other counties of the State, the general paralysis occasioned by the Yellow Fever epidemic and attendant quarantine regulations . . . prevented anything like a full vote being polled."[71] Additionally, the *New York Herald* in its November 7 edition listed congressional election results, reporting that "on the west side of the state the vote is light, in consequence of the epidemic and quarantine." The reporter continued by stating that all Democrats had been reelected, and he wrote that in the capital city of Jackson only twenty-seven votes were cast in the election.[72]

Some cities that did legislate and enforce strict quarantines, however, did not escape the epidemic. Just as Holly Springs's officials were unrestricted in their decision-making process, so too were other locales' health officers. The cities of Greenwood and Water Valley both provide good examples of strict quarantines. Both of these locations established and made efforts to enforce tight quarantine restrictions through local action as they attempted to stymie yellow fever's advance into their communities.

On August 13, Greenwood officials passed a quarantine ordinance that "prohibited [all persons] from entering the corporate limits of the town . . . under penalty of *One Hundred and Fifty Dollars* until the first day of October, unless they can show that they are not from any locality infected with Yellow Fever and that they have not traveled on steamboat or railroad within ten days of their *entrance* into said town." Officials hoped that the steep fine would deter anyone from breaking the quarantine lines around Greenwood, not realizing that more than likely the town was already infected. As the number of deaths mounted in the city, volunteers enforcing the lines were unable to guard the city limits and perform their duties because of stretched manpower.[73]

The experience of Water Valley, forty-eight miles south of Holly Springs, is also instructive regarding the ineffectiveness of quarantine regulations. Prior to the yellow fever epidemic, Water Valley was a town of approximately three thousand, about half African American and half white. Its health officials established quarantines after the first case of yellow fever appeared in the city. Ironically, once the first case appears, it is too late for quarantines. Kenny Lees, a railroad worker, was the first citizen in Water Valley to contract and succumb to the fever. When knowledge of a yellow fever death became public, panic usually prevailed. One account stated that people began "refugeeing" immediately out of Water Valley, leaving the town in "the greatest terror and confusion."[74] Citizens usually left as quickly as possible after yellow fever's appearance because they wanted to avoid any quarantine restrictions that would make travel difficult or impossible. Therefore, after the initial panicked rush out of town Water Valley counted only about five hundred remaining citizens, most of whom were African Americans. Soon thereafter, local quarantines were the order of business around Water Valley. Those citizens who did not possess the means to flee the town were left to cope behind the quarantine lines. Because of economic difficulties, African Americans in particular experienced this problem.

As part of Water Valley's quarantine restrictions, all northbound trains on the Illinois Central Railroad line were prohibited. However, officials allowed trains carrying mail and passengers to stop one mile south of the city in order to unload mail and allow travelers with proper health certificates to disembark and whose destination was Water Valley and the surrounding countryside. Health officials believed that situating a stop a mile away could keep yellow fever contagion out of their city as they inspected individuals and potential fomite carriers at that distant location. After discharging its "legal" cargo, officials then allowed the train to proceed through the town with the remainder of its passengers and cargo at a speed of forty miles per hour, provided all doors and windows were locked. Perhaps officials believed also that if any yellow fever contagion did exist on the train, it could not land in their city if the train was going fast enough. Regardless of these efforts at enforcing quarantines, the restrictions around Water Valley were ineffective because possibly viremic refugees from Grenada (and mosquitoes) evaded the quarantine guards and entered the city, thus spreading the disease.[75]

Health officials in Water Valley also implemented the state board of health's recommended guidelines throughout the city by dispensing lime and carbolic acid for disinfection. The Chicago, St. Louis and New Orleans Railroad had donated a carload of lime to Water Valley for this purpose and possibly to create an atmosphere of goodwill so that it could maintain rail service through the town's limits. City officials also ordered the burning of pine knots or torches in the street to drive away yellow fever "miasma." Many officials and common folk believed that the thick smoke from burning sap-rich pine warded off any yellow fever "bad air." Quarantine restrictions, disinfectants, and burning pine were all commonly recommended methods of preventing an outbreak of yellow fever. The state board of health also endorsed these actions as local citizens assumed control of their own health measures.[76]

In spite of diligent preventive efforts, Water Valley officials declared a yellow fever epidemic on August 15. Most of those who initially contracted the disease were white males who worked for the Chicago, St. Louis and New Orleans Railroad or the local telegraph company. The president of the Yalobusha County Board of Health reported that yellow fever cases in Water Valley were most virulent among white males who drank excessively: "It was very fatal with persons of irregular habits of all kinds, but especially with those addicted to regular drinking." The same health official also noted that the "disease was in general mild and easily controlled among the Negroes, many of them getting well without scarcely any treatment at all."[77] Given some contemporary treatment methods, perhaps African Americans were recovering in Water Valley simply because they did not receive medical treatment from white physicians. Historically, African Americans usually preferred to manage their own medical problems through herbal home remedies rather than subjecting themselves to harsh white prescriptives and racial prejudice.[78]

Quarantine restrictions also severely interrupted business in Water Valley. Reports abounded that guards in the city along the restrictive boundaries had shot people who attempted to trespass the lines. However, extensive research did not unearth any such incident. The panic of the epidemic more than likely created an atmosphere tense with uncertainty and rife with rumors. The fear of encountering shotgun-armed quarantine guards certainly hindered commercial activity in Water Valley as Mississippians wrestled with the fearful mystery of yellow fever's appearance.

Quarantine regulations were not necessarily an effective means of yellow fever control. First and foremost, regulations were almost useless against the *Aedes aegypti* mosquito, the vector. The chances of excluding that first infected person traveling to a community were slim at best. Sadly for 1878 Mississippians, they had no sound knowledge of yellow fever transmission. Also, even if citizens had been cognizant of the mode of transmission, individual towns were not legally bound to establish and enforce any intrastate travel restrictions to and from yellow fever areas. Villages, towns, and cities were dependent upon individual initiative. The Mississippi State Board of Health could only suggest the creation of quarantines; it could not mandate restrictions. As a result, quarantine boundaries and quarantine enforcement were arbitrary. In this uncontrolled situation, rumors such as those in Water Valley regarding shotgun quarantines flourished. Moreover, if quarantine lines were established and adequately maintained, their effectiveness was often compromised by people sneaking through or around them in search of that elusive safe haven. Mississippians were determined to seek safety and were willing to risk personal security and disregard local authorities as they took their chances running the quarantine lines.

Another effort to offer some peace of mind to Mississippians was Governor John M. Stone's proclamation recommending a statewide day of prayer that should be observed for all fever-stricken communities. Stone declared September 30, 1878, the official day of prayer for all Mississippians. Citizens in the state were distressed as the plague continued unabated across the state. As a contemporary noted, "Once again since the terrible war between the States, towns and cities will be found depopulated, family circles broken up, homes desolated and darkened, and business demoralized and destroyed. God grant there may never come another such [as the epidemic of 1878]."[79] On September 27 the proclamation appeared throughout Mississippi in those newspapers still operating. Stone stated, "Whereas, the hand of affliction has been laid heavily upon our people, and a fearful epidemic is prevailing in many portions of the state . . . and no relief has been found in human skill . . . I . . . do recommend that . . . all Christian people throughout the State repair to their respective places of worship and offer up their united petition in prayer to God, that he will withdraw from our people this terrible affliction . . . and that He . . . will restore them to health and bring peace to their mourning households." Stone neglected to be inclusive in his planned prayer day, however. The Jewish citizens of Natchez telegraphed the governor, asking, "On what day will the Jews be permitted to offer up Thanksgiving since the thierteeth [sic] set as day for Christians." Evidence does not reveal the exact day decided upon for the Jewish community in Natchez and other Mississippi locales. More than likely, Mississippians of all religious persuasions appealed daily to a higher power as yellow fever sustained its grip across the state.

Even though Stone's proclamation appeared to be an earnest gesture of concern, not all Mississippians were satisfied with the governor's suggestion, and several newspaper editors printed criticisms. The *Jackson Clarion* suggested that, instead of praying, the state legislators should appropriate $100,000 for relief efforts. The *Pascagoula Democrat-Star* editorialized that although prayer was good, "what the people in the infected districts need is money and supplies, and although appeals have been responded to liberally from all parts of the Union it is none the less a duty of the State to contribute to the relief of distress within our own limits." Many thought that an extra session of the legislature was necessary to appropriate money "for the relief of the destitution which now exists. Our citizens should not be compelled to call upon others outside of the State for aid as long as there is a dollar in Mississippi, and we see no impropriety in the governor convening the legislature for the purpose of extending relief to the citizens of the State." The editors of the *Democrat-Star* closed by stating that the governor "had entirely ignored the wishes of the people of the State." The editor of the *Aberdeen Examiner* penned a more vitriolic response, stating that the prayer proclamation was "pitiful" and a "poor response to the general demand for him to exercise his power and influence for the relief of a suffering people who should not need outside aid, and do not wish to be humiliated by having to accept it." Prayers were "ascending at morn, noon, and night, from every household," the *Examiner*'s editor maintained, and Stone should exercise his executive power to "use public resources for the public good" rather than worry about prayer fulfillments.[80]

However, the exact parameters of what defined state intervention were never clearly outlined. Just as with the New Orleans and Memphis epidemics, citizens' demands for state intervention generally rested upon quarantine issues and not upon the use of public resources. Locales in all three states demanded assistance with combating the spread of intra- and interstate disease. During this crisis, citizens needed a strong government presence assisting them as they attempted to deal with the demands of the epidemic, but the state legislatures were not adequately empowered to do so. In fact, it would not be until after the 1878 epidemic that the national government would address expanded health care issues and quarantine regulations chiefly in the South. Until that occurred, the states depended largely upon local charities like the Howard Association and outside sources of provisions and monetary aid. This self-reliance ultimately helped to fashion the consciousness of public health in Mississippi and other southern states.

Without official state intervention, civic officials assumed their paternalistic responsibilities and began to mobilize health measures within the confines of their towns during the opening weeks of the epidemic. Medical officials and hastily created local health boards quickly enacted sanitary measures and controls for their respective regions, as the state board of health could not. From the Mississippi State Board of Health, Johnston created a blueprint for the state's local officials to follow, but many locales chose not to use it. Bureaucrats in Water Valley adhered to Johnston's suggestions, however, so their actions exemplified sanitary controls recommended by the state board of health. Certainly, self-government was evident in the initial stage of the epidemic.

By the end of August 1878, Mississippians had only begun to experience the harsh effects of yellow fever.[81] Mortality rates began to climb, and commerce slowed. Quarantine lines were arbitrary at best, Mississippians were dying, and businesses were beginning to feel the stress of shortages. The events of July and August merely hinted at the challenges ahead, and the state was unprepared for the difficult times to come.

4
Responses to Yellow Fever

It seemed as if hell had been moved up on earth.
—*Frank Leslie's Illustrated Newspaper,* September 1878

In September 1878, business operations screeched to a halt as quarantine lines enveloped many of Mississippi's municipalities. Life became a waiting game for yellow fever, and the mounting death toll disheartened and alarmed citizens throughout the state. Under these circumstances, Mississippians found that their newly reconstructed government could provide little by way of help or comfort as quarantines made life more difficult without halting the disease. The government, elected on a platform of self-reliance, reinforced the sense that individuals and communities were on their own. At the same time, though, this was not antebellum Mississippi. It was a state in transition, in which much local paternalism had broken down in self-interest, and whose citizens, white and, particularly, black, had more expectation of help. Charities, both local and national, stepped in to fill the vacuum, but this clearly highlighted the need for real government involvement.

The Mississippi State Board of Health could only offer advice and request statistics as the epidemic progressed. However, the president pro tem, the secretary of the board, and several of its members, acting on their own, suggested to Governor Stone that a 50 percent cut in the telegraph service rate would help relieve Mississippians of some economic stress.[1] This effort was not a board motion—it reflected the helplessness some members felt in their efforts to aid fellow citizens. County boards of health, created under the state board's auspices, had little power to prosecute individuals who disregarded local health regulations.

Making the failure of the government even more blatant, the majority of the affected locations experienced an overwhelming loss of the civic personnel who would have performed those prosecutorial duties. City employees had either contracted the disease or had fled. For instance, on August 22 four members of Grenada's relief committee had informed Governor Stone that no "civil officer of any kind" was in that city: "Our sheriff & city marshall and their deputies are dead or gone. Our mayor is dead—and but one of the Board of Alderman left & he [is] sick—our population is reduced to the sick, the doctors, nurses & undertakers—our people generally have fled the city." The committee members further informed the governor that because fellow citizens had left in great numbers, businesses were left unattended and "exposed to thieves & burglers [*sic*]. They have commenced their work already. There are a few desperate characters here and they are reduced to desperate straits." The four committee members requested a "police force" to avoid "serious difficulties," as they had "no parallel in the history of yellow fever to the suferings [*sic*] and mortality that has been upon us. We are in the midst of death." They closed by stating, "Help us if you can." No confirmation exists whether Governor Stone was able to allay the relief committee's worries. Many communities were simply left to their own administrative devices during the epidemic months.[2] It is also clear from the letter that many locales were simply not up to the task, creating a veritable vacuum of local government.

Frustration was clearly mounting when on September 9 Dr. J. D. McRae in Grenada sent a letter to Stone in which he outlined the situation there and begged for assistance. He confirmed that the mayor of Grenada had died three weeks earlier and that the city's marshal and the entire board of aldermen had "left for the country or are dead." Thieves had already robbed three houses in Grenada, and the remaining citizens found themselves at their mercy. A temporary mayor could "alleviate some of the horrors of our deplorable condition," and Dr. McRae tendered his services to fill that position, "believing that every one should do all he can to alleviate human misery." However, the mayoral appointment was not forthcoming, as Stone replied, "your appointment would have no legal power to either remove nuisances or organizing a night watch, as the city would not be bound to pay any necessary expense for any such purpose."[3] The governor's power was so limited as to be useless, and Stone made no visible effort to encroach on the town's rights—even when he was begged to do so.

To fill the vacuum, private relief organizations and committees took responsibility for aiding those areas stricken by yellow fever. Relief committees throughout the state began mobilizing in August, and by September their operations were well under way. Regardless of these earnest relief efforts, the situation in Mississippi during the epidemic remained dreadful. By September, no absolutely safe havens existed in the state.

Charitable organizations had existed in Mississippi before the 1878 yellow fever epidemic. The Order of Sisters of Charity already had a long history of helping the people of Holly Springs. During the Civil War they had attended wounded Confederate soldiers there, and in 1868 they established Bethlehem Academy, a Catholic school for girls in Holly Springs with an original enrollment of fifty.[4] This sort of charity transcended the state's political seesaw. In the late nineteenth century, Catholic nursing orders had proliferated, as had their Protestant counterparts. What is striking in 1878 Mississippi is the degree to which they had to take charge in the absence of effective government at any level.

Another major charitable organization compensating for health deficiencies in 1878 Mississippi was a group of volunteers calling themselves the Howards. The group first commenced operations in New Orleans as the Young Men's Howard Association when a group of thirty civic-minded men organized this charitable society after the 1837 yellow fever epidemic there. Named after British philanthropist John Howard (1726–90), the group was nonsectarian and treated anyone, particularly the indigent, regardless of race, color, or sex. Separate facilities existed for whites and blacks, but the Howards provided the necessary medical personnel and provisions to all. For example, in Canton a separate hospital for black yellow fever victims was established during the epidemic. The Howards relied exclusively upon donations to accomplish their relief work among the sick and poor populace. Incorporated on February 28, 1842, the Howards, as they came to be known, obtained a state charter from Louisiana and began traveling to locations that suffered yellow fever and cholera outbreaks, offering help and relief aid. Thereafter, any locally created benevolent organization that focused particularly on yellow fever relief work assumed the name Howard Association. The Howards did not change as a result of the Civil War. Their vision remained steadfast and completely separate from government. During the 1878 yellow fever epidemic, Howard associations sprang up throughout the South.[5] The Howards arranged for physicians and nurses to travel to locales with yellow fever and provide medical care. The organization hired nursing personnel apparently without regard to gender or race. Often the nurses and doctors were from areas outside the epidemic's epicenter. With nursing care and all necessities provided by the Howards, most of the victims whom they treated survived.

The Order of Freemasons also proved to be a godsend. Their fundamental commitment to benevolence and donations for the relief of distressed widows and orphans provided a constant source of aid and comfort to many victims of the yellow fever epidemic.[6] Often working with the Howards in 1878, Freemasons from forty-one states and territories donated money to cities across Mississippi. As J. L. Power, the grand secretary of Freemasons in Mississippi, stated, "a Mason's charity should be as extensive as the wants of suffering humanity."[7]

Because of their past experiences in yellow fever epidemics, Mississippians expected help from charitable organizations during the 1878 epidemic. Yellow fever epidemics had raged regularly in the state prior to the 1878 outbreak. For example, in 1847 the *New Orleans Daily Picayune* called for charitable associations to organize in order to tend citizens stricken with yellow fever in the city and along the Mississippi Gulf Coast: "It may be unnecessary, but cannot be improper, to call upon the young men . . . who are familiar with the disease, to revive those charitable associations which in former years have saved so many lives and mitigated so much anguish."[8] The paper reported that the Howards had organized relief efforts for New Orleans and the coast, affirming that "In times past the Association [Howards] has been infinitely useful. We feel confident that it will maintain its reputation this season."[9] The *Daily Picayune* also included the Masons in a list of sources titled "Medical Aid for the Poor."[10] Advertisements and editorials appear throughout the antebellum years, calling for relief organizations to provide aid to the suffering.

Private and parochial charities also operated throughout the epidemic months in 1878, providing provisions and medical and financial aid to stricken citizens. In addition, smaller charitable efforts such as local musical performances contributed much-needed cash to hometown folks. Private individuals also collected money and goods nationwide as the yellow fever continued to spread throughout the fall. Mississippians benefited from the aid these sundry organizations and charity drives provided, as the state was unable to offer relief to its stricken citizens.

The town of Holly Springs provides an excellent case study both of what worked and what did not work in a crisis managed by a patchwork of charities and local self-help. In early September, as news spread of refugee deaths in Holly Springs, the majority of the town's citizens fled to safer locations. According to Helen Craft Anderson, "Men, women and children struggled in one mighty effort as the first flight from the presence of an unseen foe. Trunks were packed hastily with such articles as came nearest to hand." As the alarm continued throughout the first week of September, "the streets leading to the depot were crowded, while every available vehicle was filled with baggage and human beings in one confused rush of frantic fear lest the outgoing train should leave them, and every moment of detention had in it the tick of death." This scene of mass confusion occurred throughout Mississippi as citizens boarded trains to any destination outside yellow fever's perimeters. In Holly Springs and elsewhere, the refugees included most "leading citizens" and "pillars of the community"— the only insiders able to mobilize effective relief. Those who stayed were the "sick, the dying, the poor who could not leave, and the few who would not."[11]

Those who stayed in Holly Springs after the mass exodus found comfort in charity, not in government. Some had remained out of a sense of duty. These local health officials and volunteers remaining to care for yellow fever victims quickly requisitioned the Marshall County Courthouse and turned it into a hospital. The beds for yellow fever patients consisted of simple straw piles that could be easily removed when they became soiled. Community help was not sufficient, though, and outside charity came to take up some of the slack. From Nazareth, Kentucky, twelve Sisters of Charity quickly established a nursing station at the makeshift hospital with Father Anacletus Oberti, the local priest from St. Joseph's Catholic Church, directing them.[12] There was nothing new in their presence as residents were familiar with the Sisters of Charity and Sisters of Mercy outreach programs.[13]

While some patients were fortunate to be nursed at home by family members, others had to rely upon the kindness of strangers. These volunteers exhibited remarkable devotion toward their patients. At the courthouse hospital the Sisters of Charity labored long hours under the guidance of Howard Association doctors, many of whom were from outside Mississippi. One author described the sisters' work in the following manner: "Like angels of mercy, they hovered over the loathsome spot day and night, caring not who the patient might be if only his life could be spared. One by one these sisters fell until six of them, with the faithful priest, Father Oberti, lay dead."[14] A single monument marks their collective grave in Holly Springs. Dr. Swearingen, the Howard Association doctor who worked alongside the sisters at the courthouse hospital, was so moved by Sister Corinthia's devotion to her patients that he scratched a tribute to her on a wall in the courthouse hospital following her death:

Within this room September 1878 Sister Corintha [sic] sank into sleep eternal among the first to enter this realm of death. She was the last save one to leave. The writer of this humble notice saw her in health gentle but strong as she moved with noiseless steps and serene smiles through the crowded wards. He saw her when the yellow plumed angel threw his golden shadows over the last sad scene and eye unused to weeping payed [sic] the tribute of tears to the brave and beautiful 'Spirit of Mercy.'

> She needs no slab of parian marble
> With its white and ghastly head.
> To tell wanderers in the valley
> The virtues of the dead.
> Let the lily be her tombstone
> And dew drops pure and bright,
> The epitaphs the Angels write
> In the stillness of the night.
> R. M. Swearingen, M. D.
> Austin, Texas
> *Let no one deface this.*[15]

The Sisters of Charity stationed at the courthouse hospital labored unceasingly to nurse the sick and dying, black and white. According to the *History of Marshall County, Mississippi,* they "took charge of the main hospital and did not shrink from anything and did not spare themselves from the work of mercy."[16]

Drs. F. W. Dancy and William McCorkle Compton, members of the state board of health and residents of Holly Springs, urged a strict city quarantine in late August, but the mayor and aldermen overruled them in early September. The "City of Flowers" maintained its policy of sanctuary and "opened wide its gates as a city of refuge to all who might come there," while the Sisters of Charity toiled in the hospital. Out of a population of approximately 3,500, only about 1,500 citizens remained in the city after the initial mass evacuation. Of course, those remaining residents, 300 whites and 1,200 African Americans, along with the religious order, were the ones who welcomed and cared for refugees arriving from surrounding areas.[17]

The citizens of Holly Springs also created their own relief committee, offering medical aid and provisions to locals suffering with yellow fever. Those who volunteered to serve on the committee were civic-minded individuals who were socially and politically prominent in the city. They represented the power elite in the area after Reconstruction—or at least as many as had not fled. Serving as chairman of the relief committee was Colonel W. J. L. Holland, an ex-Confederate officer. Holland was also the editor of the *Holly Springs Reporter.* The committee's secretary was another ex-Confederate officer, Captain Thomas B. Rogers.[18]

Together with the Sisters of Charity and Father Oberti, the newly created relief committee appealed to the Howard Association for aid in the first week of September. After September 4, when Holly Springs' health officials declared that yellow fever was epidemic in that city, doctors, nurses, a telegraph operator, druggists, and assistants began arriving from the New Orleans Howards. One of them reported to the grand secretary of Masons via Western Union telegram on September 5 that the yellow fever was "bad" in Holly Springs and Greenville. That same day, a telegram from Holly Springs to Governor Stone pleaded, "For God's sake send us some nurses and doctors. All down with fever. We are destitute." It should be clear by now which organizations responded with effective aid. It is only fair to note that the state faced severe financial problems, the legacy of the war years and Reconstruction, but it also lacked the political will to act.[19] Therefore, it is not surprising that the governor's office did not fulfill the request. However, on September 13 the Howards in New Orleans alerted the Holly Springs Relief Committee that ten more nurses were on their way to their city. The Howards also informed city officials that if they required other vital supplies, that organization would send them upon request. Dr. B. F. McKie, a local physician, and Dr. Compton of the state board of health also remained in Holly Springs to help nurse the sick.[20]

Why did so many local community leaders believe that the state government would help? Had they not voted for this new Democratic government, which ran on a platform of self-reliance? The state had played a minimal role in epidemic relief before the Civil War, but it can be argued that two important things had changed: first, suffering of local elites and the expectation that they are obligated to take matters in hand; and second, loathe it though they might, Reconstruction had presented a model of more active government.

The remaining residents of Holly Springs were extremely grateful to the Howard Association for sending and sponsoring medical personnel who were acclimated to the rigors of a yellow fever epidemic. Additionally, monetary relief began pouring into the city. Numerous inter- and intrastate donors made contributions to the Mississippi Masons for the relief of stricken areas. The Masons then distributed the monies through the local Howard Association or Masonic representative in each locale. By September 20, Holly Springs' remaining citizens had received approximately four thousand dollars through these relief disbursements. Beneficiaries used monetary aid in numerous ways, including purchasing medicine and food, paying doctor bills and funeral expenses, and caring for children orphaned by the epidemic.[21]

Relief aid did not alter the fact, however, that Holly Springs had never experienced yellow fever to any great extent and that local doctors were ill equipped to manage the overwhelming consequences of this disease. Many citizens in Holly Springs hailed the Howard volunteers who had come from surrounding states as heroes, and others in the city would no doubt have suffered immeasurably more during September if local doctors had been their only source of care. In fact, the local physicians themselves were susceptible to the contagion. Before September ended, the names of some Holly Springs physicians, both Howards and native, appeared in the daily death reports.[22]

The problem with volunteerism, though, is often a lack of oversight. Not all volunteers were equally responsible. For example, Dr. C. Happoldt, a fifty-two-year-old physician from North Carolina, did not fulfill his duty as expected. In a letter to Governor Stone, Governor Z. B. Vance of North Carolina stated that Happoldt, a seasoned yellow fever health professional, had been in Memphis in 1873, so he knew the necessary treatments for yellow fever. However, Happoldt was an "intemperate man" and had taken the travel money given to him by an aid society and used it to get drunk instead of departing to Mississippi to help yellow fever victims. Vance stated that Happoldt was "worthless" but "really eminent in his profession, especially in treating yellow fever."[23]

Some nurses, too, behaved with a distinct lack of propriety. For instance, the

Howards recruited a group of nurses from Washington, D.C., to tend to southerners stricken with yellow fever. While traveling south, the nurses reportedly engaged in "the most reckless style of kissing and hugging on the [railroad] cars after leaving Louisville," and "decent people" observed "an event approaching the most abandoned exploits of bacchanals" on the platform of a Pullman sleeper near Colesburg, Kentucky. These "naughty nurses" continued to drink champagne and indulge in "promiscuous love-making" for the duration of the trip, at one time even dancing "around a whiskey bottle like Indians."[24]

While those traveling nurses seem to have simply gotten out of hand, wrongdoing of a more calculated sort also appeared. As W. J. L. Holland of the Holly Springs Relief Committee reported, an assistant male nurse from Martin, Tennessee, named S. Thomas robbed a patient under the care of Mrs. Laborde, the head nurse. When law officers arrested Thomas, he attempted to swallow the money rather than be caught with the evidence. His trick did not work, however, and officials locked him in the Holly Springs jail. Mrs. Laborde worried that all of the excitement would cause her patient to relapse.[25]

The epidemic also demonstrated that reliance on a sense of duty alone was not adequate in an emergency of this scope. Dereliction of duty and irresponsibility were not confined to the incoming professionals, as Mississippians themselves sometimes behaved in a less than stellar manner. For example, Dr. Warren Stone of New Orleans complained that locals in Grenada would not provide regular meals to the Howard doctors because there was not a "single black or white man or woman who would take charge of the culinary department." The kitchen facilities for the physicians were in the Chamberlain House, and owing to the number of sick and dying patients hospitalized there, no townsperson would enter the home to cook. Additionally, Stone reported that doctors did not have enough vehicles to use for their house visits around Grenada. In fact, as reported in the *New York Herald,* wagons were unavailable in that city for many necessary purposes, including funerals.[26] Burying the dead became a problem around the state as the yellow fever spread.

Self-help was often the last resort of desperate people. Further west, J. E. Becton, a master railroad mechanic and resident of Water Valley, reported that he could not recruit anyone to help him bury Kenney Lees, a local yellow fever victim. Reverting to self-help, Becton buried Lees and, with the help of local "railroad boys," guarded Lees's house after others threatened to burn it, believing that fire would kill any yellow fever remaining on the premises. The failure of any government intervention resulted in a reversion to vigilante-style self-defense, just as when organizations such as the Ku Klux Klan had taken matters into their own hands during Reconstruction. Guarding the premises, the railroad workers "gave the cowardly firebugs a warm reception with buckshot and powder" when they attempted to destroy the home. However, actions outside the moral boundaries of nineteenth-century expectations were far rarer than instances of heroics. The majority of those who chose to remain in fever-stricken regions understood that "there was nothing but hard work for all who, with any conscience at all, endeavor to perform their duty to the general weal and their own satisfaction," and therefore remained at their posts valiantly.[27]

Although many Mississippians offered their services unselfishly, citizens had no choice but to rely upon volunteers, most of them from other states, to combat the effects of this epidemic. In doing so, the state created a double-edged situation. The volunteers from organizations like the Howards brought with them needed manpower and provisions such as medicines because Mississippi was clearly unable to care for its own and therefore had to rely upon outside help. With a state board of health that had no legislative power and little monetary backing, Mississippi found itself completely helpless in an epidemic of this magnitude. Fortunately for Mississippians and other southerners affected by the epidemic, those organizations that buttressed the South throughout this epidemic were sincerely interested in helping those in dire need.

On September 26 the Holly Springs Relief Committee chairman reported that "The situation is growing worse. The hospital is full, and it looks like every man must go down. Only 10 out of the first 100 cases live. Two days ago, 30 new cases and 10 deaths; yesterday, 23 new cases and 11 deaths. After having recruited 5 times, the Relief Committee yesterday numbered 1. Five hundred persons now lie stricken. We pray for friends and frost." Holland was the only member of the relief committee who was still functioning. The situation in Holly Springs was dire. "Entire families, some of them numbering eight or ten, are down with the disease," he recorded. "Among the physicians ten have been stricken down, four of these have died." Additionally, three "druggists," two ministers, and two postal workers "are in the cemetery." The victims of Yellow Jack could not be buried fast enough, and rows of "ghastly" coffins lined the courthouse lawn "waiting for the ghastlier bodies. . . . The only sound, other than those in the cemetery, to shatter the stillness of the night, is the dismal howling of dogs, making a gruesome requiem for the dead."[28]

Efforts to gain assistance from public and charitable organizations should not blind us to the most fundamental response to disease—the care family members gave to each other in the face of almost certain death. This is an issue that goes far beyond politics or even southern culture. Abnormal situations resulted from the stress of the epidemic, and those who remained behind quarantine lines often experienced unusual circumstances. Under these horrible conditions people moved beyond ordinary, expected standards of behavior. For instance, in some cases, uninfected family members, safe in other locales from the yellow fever contagion, returned to an infected region to care for family members trapped behind quarantine lines.

One such person was Katharine Bonner McDowell, an author of southern tales who wrote under the pseudonym Sherwood Bonner. She was from Holly Springs, and her family was part of that city's aristocracy. She therefore had led a privileged life while growing up. By 1878, however, she had left her husband and young child to pursue an education and career in Boston. While she was in Boston honing her writing skills, Henry Wadsworth Longfellow befriended her and became her mentor and patron. Regardless of this new life far from the perils of plague-stricken Holly Springs, McDowell, upon reading about the city's yellow fever in the Boston press and receiving urgent letters from family and friends, decided to return home to help her daughter, Lilian, and other family members who remained behind quarantine lines. She hoped to convince her father and brother to leave Holly Springs and join her mother and sisters in Kentucky.[29]

McDowell encountered several problems while attempting to reach Holly Springs. She had to wait two days in Cincinnati to catch the southbound train that traveled into Mississippi, as we know from her ongoing correspondence with Longfellow throughout her arduous trip south. The scene that greeted McDowell when she finally entered Holly Springs on September 2 shocked her. The town was eerily quiet, as most citizens had already fled ahead of the yellow fever. Those who did stay expressed dismay, expecting the worst at any moment.[30]

Two days after McDowell arrived, Colonel A. W. Goodrich, a former mayor of Holly Springs, became the first casualty of yellow fever. McDowell urged her father, Dr. Charles Bonner, to leave the city with her brother, Samuel, and to take Lilian and her aunt Martha to a safe location. Mrs. Bonner and McDowell's two sisters were safe in Kentucky and were anxious for the other family members to join them. However, Dr. Bonner and Samuel refused to leave town, feeling it their duty to aid those who remained behind. McDowell's brother had no medical training, yet he chose to stay and help his father aid others. McDowell decided then to send her daughter with her aunt Martha unescorted to Penn Yan, New York, for their safety. By this time, she had also decided to remain in Holly Springs and help her father and brother nurse the yellow fever victims.[31]

Two days later, on September 4, McDowell's father and brother contracted yellow fever. McDowell wired Longfellow regarding this dire situation that day, beseeching, "Help for God's sake. Send money. Father & brother down [with] yellow fever. Alone to nurse." The next day she again telegraphed Longfellow, lamenting that "My heart [is] breaking. Fear I have the fever."[32]

On September 7, McDowell's father and brother died of yellow fever. Citizens quickly buried their bodies in deep graves along with those of other victims. Two days later, McDowell, with the help of friends, broke through the newly established Holly Springs quarantine and returned to Cincinnati. She had not, despite her fear, contracted yellow fever. From Cincinnati she wired Longfellow: "father & brother dead, Just arrived here well but wearied. Your check with miscarried baggage. Please telegraph the amount today." Longfellow apparently wired money to her as soon as he could, for another telegram from McDowell arrived at his house that same day: "Money received. No more needed, and trying to reach Boston."[33]

McDowell returned to Holly Springs in November 1878 to finalize her family's affairs. Her second trip was fraught with as much sadness as the first. No family members greeted her when she arrived in the city, as her mother, sisters, aunt, and daughter were still refugees in New York. No dear friends welcomed her, thanks to Bronze John (yellow fever). McDowell wrote to Longfellow from Holly Springs on November 28, "I am at home again—if this great desolate house can be called home. . . . I have cried until my eyes hurt so they cannot bear the light." As Hubert H. McAlexander has stated, "The fever cut across her life and marked the end of a prolonged youth."[34]

In Holly Springs, the experiences of the Wells family mirrored that of the Bonners. Both families were closely knit and involved in religious and political organizations in the city. However, they differed in that the Wells family was African American. In 1878, James and Elizabeth Wells lived in the city with their eight children, four boys and four girls, one of whom was Ida Bell, whom we have to thank for her account of the epidemic. Both James and Elizabeth had been slaves—James a carpenter, Elizabeth a cook. Upon emancipation, the Wellses renewed their wedding vows in a Christian ceremony. James then became politically active in the Loyal League, a Republican political organization, while his wife and children attended Shaw University in Holly Springs to learn to read and write. By 1878 the family appeared to be situated well in the black community of Holly Springs.[35]

When yellow fever appeared in Holly Springs, the sixteen-year-old Ida was in the countryside near the city, visiting her grandmother. Her family urged her to remain there as the city suffered the epidemic. Like McDowell, however, Ida risked her personal safety to be with her stricken family. She later stated in her autobiography that "the conviction grew within me that I ought to be with them. . . . There's nobody but me to look after them now."[36] Perhaps she knew that because of the racial strife of post-Reconstruction Mississippi, her family and other African Americans would not be the first to receive aid from any organized benevolent society. She therefore returned to Holly Springs and nursed her father, mother, and one sibling after they had contracted yellow fever.

On September 26, James Wells died of yellow fever. His wife succumbed the next day. On October 3, "Jim Well's child (colored)" also died of the disease, as recorded by J. L. Power. The deaths of James and Elizabeth Wells are also listed in Keating's *History of the Yellow Fever*.[37] No contemporary sources contain grand descriptions of this couple or lengthy praise of their contributions to Holly Springs comparable to those dedicated to the Bonners. However, both families exemplified strong family ties and the loyalty of their daughters.

The experiences of Katharine Bonner McDowell and Ida Wells reflect the prevailing situation in Mississippi at the time. Neither family expected help from government as the daughters made arrangements for their family members' health care and burial. Although the Bonners would have had more access to organized charity, they preferred to be independent, while the Wellses had little if any say in the matter. These two families emphasized self-help and independence, whether by choice or necessity.

In Holly Springs and other towns throughout Mississippi, citizens coped with the ravages of yellow fever as best they could. People often risked their own lives to nurse their kin. Yellow fever crossed all economic boundaries in 1878, even affecting families in prestigious political positions. For example, Holly Springs native Kinloch Falconer, Mississippi's secretary of state, was also a victim of the disease. He was in Jackson when news came that the plague had appeared in his hometown. His family had deep connections to Holly Springs; at one time Falconer had been the editor of the *Holly Springs Reporter,* and he was mayor of that city before his election to state office. Later, he and his brother, Howard, had established a law practice in Holly Springs prior to Falconer's election; therefore, his ties to the city were economic as well as familial. Falconer went "right into the jaws of death" when he returned home to nurse his dying father and sick brother. He asked Governor Stone to appoint an interim secretary of state before he hurried home to aid his kinfolk. Falconer nursed and then buried his father and brother shortly after his return to Holly Springs. While engaged in their health care, he too "was smitten with the plague," and he died on September 23. Local papers described him as "a true gentleman" and one of Mississippi's "best and truest sons."[38]

Living up to the nineteenth-century ideal of southern manhood, Kinloch Falconer had not hesitated to return to Holly Springs to nurse his family during this epidemic. He represented an ideal of southern manhood. He doubtless would have gone to nurse his family in Holly Springs even if government agencies had been providing more effective help—that being one of the positive sides of independent southern patriarchy—and probably would have died under any circumstances. But his death and the way Mississippi society commemorated it made him one of the many icons of old southern values, helping to drive home the point that the new government dispensation was correct.[39]

Newspapers across Mississippi eulogized Falconer. One stated, "Thus has passed away in the zenith of splendid manhood, one of Mississippi's grandest sons, doubly a hero, heroic in war's carnage, grandly heroic in the carnival pestilence." The *American Citizen* of Canton praised Falconer as "noble and chivalric" as he "had fallen before the relentless scythe of death."[40] The praise heaped upon Falconer not only recognized his contribution to Holly Springs but also validated the notion that individual action was most important in this crisis, both because government intervention was sorely lacking and because self-reliance was being idolized as a core value. In catastrophe, some people always exhibit selfless care of others. What is notable in 1878 is the way contemporary accounts acknowledged their heroism—white male heroism, that is. The recurrent belief that "we will survive because of southern values" was even applied at times to northerners.

Accounts abound of heroic efforts of caregivers during the yellow fever epidemic. For instance, the local paper hailed two brothers from Logtown in Harrison County as exceedingly brave men for their actions in that town's epidemic. Randall and Willie Stocker provided basic care to those stricken with yellow fever, untiringly nursing the sick and dying, even though they did not have any medical training. Also in that town, Dr. J. A. Mead, a twenty-seven-year-old from Lowell, Massachusetts, "stood bravely at his post and did all in his power to check the ravages of the yellow fiend." Mead was one of a host of volunteers who came south to tend to the yellow fever victims. He did not contract the disease while he cared for the citizens of Logtown.[41] The seeming paradox in Logtown is that on one hand, the yellow fever epidemic reaffirmed traditional southern values; on the other hand, the South was now a part of the greater United States. As never before, southerners had to see that at least some people from the North had "southern" virtues, too. Thus, the 1878 epidemic helped drive the wedge of eventual change further into society, even as it cemented a restored southern patriarchy into place.

The actions of charitable groups did not negate the fact that charity began at home in the 1878 epidemic. On the front lines were the religious leaders of many communities, who on the whole stayed and practiced what they preached. To return to our case of Holly Springs, as yellow fever cases and deaths rose, many religious leaders in the community found themselves in a quandary. Was it their duty to stay with their flocks and risk contracting yellow fever, or should they flee along with the majority of their congregations? For example, two Methodist ministers, J. D. Cameron and J. W. Lawrence, abandoned the city along with its fleeing citizens when they heard news of yellow fever. The editors of the *Pascagoula Democrat-Star* asked on September 13, "When the preachers are afraid of death, what is to be expected of ordinary mortals?" On the other hand, the Presbyterian, Baptist, and Catholic clergy all remained in Holly Springs for the epidemic. Sadly, records reveal that all of them contracted the fever by September 10. By then, twenty-one people had died in Holly Springs, and forty new cases of the fever had appeared. As one Holly Springs citizen lamented, "Death is making a harvest around us."[42]

Religious vows and devotion to humanity motivated many who provided aid. During the epidemic, caregivers also acted as medical consultants, hospital administrators, and, of course, empathetic listeners. Their responsibilities often spanned twenty-four-hour shifts, frequently with no relief. Many of these people died while performing their pastoral duties.

However, at least one Protestant clergyman criticized clerics when they entered patients' sickrooms not as caregivers but as heralds of death. Rev. Charles Kimball Marshall, a prominent southern Methodist minister of Vicksburg and caregiver during previous yellow fever outbreaks, expressed his admiration for members of religious orders and clergy who acted as caregivers, but he censured physicians who permitted clerics to hover over patients, awaiting their deaths. "I fully believe," Marshall asserted, "that there are not a few lying asleep in the graveyard whose end was hastened by the presence of clergymen and others, who, no matter of what denomination, have felt called to rush into sick rooms to show their sympathy and get the patient ready to die." He further asked, "Can five minutes' religious services over a poor fellow covered with blisters, choked with black vomit, and barely able to tell his nurses what he wants, . . . renovate a moral nature steeped in unbelief and sin for fifty years?"[43] Regardless of Marshall's critique, Mississippians sought the succor of their religious leaders in all stages of the disease.

Citizens of Grenada looked to H. T. Haddick, a Baptist minister, for help and inspiration during the epidemic. Haddick was away from Grenada when the fever broke out; he had fallen ill while attending a denominational convention in southern Mississippi in June. While he was recuperating, news of yellow fever in his city reached him. Disregarding his own medical needs, he "lost no time" in returning to Grenada to minister to his friends and congregation. Sadly, within two weeks of his return, Haddick "rested under the sod in the same cemetery that holds the remains of the choice members of his flock, gathered with him by the hand of the direful scourge."[44]

Rev. Charles Betts Galloway also stood bravely at his post, the Crawford Street Methodist Church in Vicksburg. Galloway and his wife chose to remain in the city to serve the sick and dying during the epidemic. Both eventually contracted the disease in September, but they recovered. The *Jackson Clarion Ledger* had erroneously reported the minister's death, and Galloway later remarked that "the death angel stayed his coming" for him. Thereafter, the pastor retained "in sacred keeping" a copy of his own obituary.[45]

In Greenville, Episcopal priest Duncan C. Green remained at St. James's Church to help yellow fever victims there. When yellow fever appeared in Greenville, he speedily dispatched his wife and two sons to the countryside while he remained behind to administer the consolations of religion and friendship. Rev. Stevenson Archer of the Presbyterian church and Rev. Tillman Page of the Methodist church also stayed in Greenville to nurse the sick and care for the dying. With the efforts of these men, "no person of any race or creed was buried without a Christian service."[46] One tribute stated that Green was "surrounded by all the sweets of domestic peace, with education, books, and refined society," and still "entered upon the untried but terrible field of labor before him." However, "in a few days he yielded up his own life, a sacrifice to humanity and Christian duty." He died on September 15. Tragically, Green did not live to see the birth of his third son on October 3. Page died a few days after Green.[47]

Soon after Green's death, Nancy Hurst Trigg organized her St. James's Sunday school class of twelve girls into a committee to honor their late priest. They earned money to purchase a marble baptismal font for the church, possibly inspired by the posthumous birth of his third son. The font was dedicated to the memory of Green; an inscription on its pedestal reads, "In Memoriam Duncan Cameron Green A Faithful Pastor 'The Good Shepherd Giveth his Life for the Sheep.'" The Young Women's Guild of St. James's Church commissioned a black walnut wood altar in Green's memory. Such tributes were not limited to his immediate community. Green's father was also a friend of Henry Wadsworth Longfellow, who, upon learning of the death of his friend's son, penned a poem as a tribute, "The Chamber Over the Gate." In that work, the poet laments the fact that an "old man [was] desolate, weeping and wailing sore for his son" whom he would see no more.[48] These two tributes obviously reflect different perspectives of Green's death. His Mississippi flock lamented the loss of a fine gentleman who performed his duty and fulfilled southern values, whereas Longfellow's rhetoric stressed the suffering that Green's father underwent when he lost his son. The tones in the two tributes vary from the southern heroic to the northern melancholic, reflecting the two societies' different emotional responses to death in the 1878 epidemic.

Nowhere, however, was the atmosphere of suspicion and fear in 1878 Mississippi clearer than in interracial relations. In most locales, dealings between African Americans and whites were further tested during the 1878 epidemic. As the disease's impact facilitated political and social restructuring into traditional antebellum ideals, the recent gains made by African Americans in Reconstruction dwindled even more as the "Redeemed" Mississippi tightened control.[49] Since the Civil War, most southern whites lived in distrust of former slaves. After the U.S. Congress voted Mississippi back into the Union on February 17, 1870, racial strife quickly developed in the state. Riots and murder occurred in cities such as Vicksburg and Clinton. According to historian Bradley Bond, "Democratic-Conservatives, who revived their party in August, 1875, . . . swore to preserve white liberty against all challengers."[50] When the violence subsided, election results revealed that the Redeemer Democrats had regained political control of Mississippi. Even in the emergency conditions of the epidemic, many politicians found it more important to put African Americans "back in their place" than to fight the disease.

To solidify their political power and to render African Americans powerless, the Democrats in August 1878 actively campaigned to maintain their hegemony. Their agenda revolved around upcoming November 5 elections and appointments to offices often vacated because of a yellow fever death. Even as Mississippi began to experience yellow fever on a grand scale, political outcomes often consumed the Democrats. Some of these decisions involved African-American Republican officeholders who demonstrated more Democratic tendencies, favoring the Democratic agenda to survive whether willingly or not. For example, Samuel McCrea, a black Republican from Greenwood, received an endorsement as voter registrar from L. P. Yerger and from another African American, Silas McLean. Yerger and McLean, interested in blocking McCrea's impending removal from office, extolled McCrea's virtues to General J. Z. George, chairman of the Democratic executive committee. They asked George to retain McCrea, describing him as "fair dealing," "conservative," and "gentlemanly in deportment," highlighting characteristics that appealed to the white conservatives and more than likely demonstrated a willingness to work with or for the Democrats. They also stressed that McCrea had made many friends "among his political enemies, the Democrats." However, McCrea possibly had difficulties fulfilling voter registration duties. His critics had stated that he was illiterate. Yerger and McLean maintained, however, that he was able to sign his name. George's decision kept McCrea in office.[51] This case helps show that the situation was by no means an absolute black versus white. However, the outlook was not good for black Mississippians.

During the growing yellow fever epidemic, African Americans began to feel economic pressures as well as political ones. For the most part, by 1878 they were dependent upon sharecropping, as were many poor whites. This agricultural system all but eliminated independent agricultural pursuits, as white and black sharecroppers, or simply "croppers," as they were called, usually only received half the income from their crops, the rest going to the landlord. For example, in 1866, W. R. Bath, a white landowner, and Ned Littlepage, a freedman, signed a sharecropping labor contract according to which Littlepage would keep one half of the cotton crop he raised, one half of the potatoes he dug, and one third of the corn and other crops he picked. Littlepage not only planted, weeded, hoed, and picked these crops on Bath's land but, as outlined in the contract, also had to harvest and store the cultivated plants and grains.[52] Moreover, open-book credit lines at local merchants often charged as much as 30 percent interest for necessary supplies, thereby creating debt that few if any could pay off. As a result, sharecroppers became dependent on the merchants as they became more indebted to the store owners. By 1875 the sharecropping system in the state had replaced one form of slavery with another.[53] Many Mississippians, therefore, were already economically stressed to the breaking point as the 1878 epidemic began, and life would become still more difficult in those regions affected by the disease as quarantine lines blocked most commercial activity.

Although the state government showed little interest or competence in helping white folk, it seemed to ignore blacks completely, except perhaps to make sure they did not get "out of line" during the crisis. The black population also had less access to organized charity. The black situation, both as givers and receivers of private assistance, shows clearly the weaknesses that hindered the development of a state health service.

As challenging politically and economically as Mississippi's environment was becoming, some humanitarian acts occurred between African Americans and whites during the 1878 yellow fever months. With a history of caregiving, African-American women demonstrated humanitarian efforts to care for whites and others during the epidemic. Noted historian of nursing Linda E. Sabin states that in the South before and during the Civil War, "while externally powerless in the world of slavery, these women [slave nurses] had considerable internal power within a family that was dependent upon them."[54] Historian Drew Gilpin Faust concludes that African-American women and men were the primary nurses during the Civil War.[55] However, any cooperation between the races during this time in Mississippi was remarkable in the light of the recent turmoil of the Reconstruction years and the Democrats' return to power.

Some African Americans remained in communities to help others, including whites, during the epidemic. Others, volunteering from different states, came to Mississippi to aid those in need. A large group of African Americans volunteered as Howard nurses to accompany James Busby Norris, a prominent white physician of Chattanooga, to Vicksburg. The Vicksburg Howards, under the guidance of President W. M. Rockwood and Secretary W. A. Fairchild, welcomed the doctor and his nurses into the city on September 3. Sixteen nurses accompanied him, including John J. Marshall (first listed as Joseph J. Marshall), Asa Peacock, Eldridge Massingale, John Johnson, Woodson Ellington, Paul Miller, John A. Logan, and Gus Williams. These nurses were all African American and may have volunteered because of the high wages being offered. They probably found the opportunity economically appealing.[56] All of the nurses were "experienced" and had already had yellow fever. On their trip to Vicksburg, the party traveled on a special train of the Alabama Great Southern Railroad line, and each nurse received a yellow-ribbon badge with "Chattanooga Yellow Fever Nurse" printed on it.[57] It is significant that 50 percent of the nurses accompanying Norris were African Americans. Were these nurses allowed to ride in the same railcars as the eight white caregivers? Did they receive some of the basketfuls of food that local Chattanooga businessmen gave to the party to tide them over on their long trip south? Under the new Democratic regime, were these African-American nurses from Tennessee treated differently than African Americans in Mississippi? Certainly these questions are pertinent, but research reveals no answers.[58] However, the spirit of volunteerism and self-sacrifice on the part of these nurses deserves attention. One contemporary wrote: "The Doctor and these nurses deserve the highest credit for the step they propose taking. They go into the midst of a plague, the ravages of which are more terrible this year than ever before. They do this for the sake of suffering humanity, risking their lives for the good of others."[59] However, no evidence exists that a white person remained in an area stricken with yellow fever to nurse African Americans in their recovery. That fact is not surprising. Newspaper accounts and personal recollections do reveal, however, appreciation for those African Americans who helped minister to others. One such example involves Bob Reed of Water Valley.

During the epidemic, Bob Reed remained in Water Valley and exemplified interracial health care efforts. Reed was an elderly African American who had assumed he was immune to yellow fever, as he had survived a previous yellow fever bout in Natchez years earlier. When officials declared a yellow fever epidemic in Water Valley, Reed began to help "both white and colored patients." He oversaw the daily nursing regimen of feeding, bathing, shaving, and administering enemas to people with the disease. He also assisted with burials. Reed's help was invaluable during the town's yellow fever epidemic because there were not enough nurses to attend to the sick after many of the town's citizens had fled. Reed demonstrated compassion during extremely troubled times.[60] He did it as a volunteer. This was not a situation of officials hiring the poor to serve as public health nurses—the state made no provision for such things.

Both African Americans and whites had to cope with horrible conditions during the epidemic, but African Americans more often bore the brunt of undue stress. For example, a black woman in Grenada had died in her home near the Chamberlain House, but the local undertaker refused to bury the corpse, which had begun to decompose. A Howard physician requisitioned a horse-and-wagon team as a hearse for the woman's burial, but townspeople surrounded the wagon and refused to allow it to proceed, an indignity unlikely to be inflicted on a white corpse. According to the account, the Howard doctor received "rough" treatment from the mob, which quickly took possession of the vehicle. Moreover, gravediggers refused to work in Grenada, so bodies often lay exposed for hours. Newspapers blamed African Americans rather than whites for the whole situation. According to a contemporary newspaper account, African Americans refused to dig graves, but they "hang around the commissary rooms, and do not miss the opportunity to receive every ration they can, whether they have had their share or not." Howards had to import gravediggers from New Orleans to help with the situation in Grenada.[61] Whether the situation was a burial or digging graves, African Americans were criticized and treated differently.

Despite the turbulent political climate, African Americans sometimes helped whites. It is logical to assume that the majority of adult African Americans living at the time of the 1878 epidemic had once been slaves. Therefore, the heroic effort demonstrated by one black woman is notable. A woman named Minerva risked her life to save two young white children in her charge. Her last name is unknown, but records indicate that before the war she had been the slave of C. Joseph Herr in Holly Springs. After the war she apparently remained with the Herr family as a house servant and nanny. When yellow fever appeared in Holly Springs, Mr. and Mrs. Herr and one of their children, an infant, contracted the disease, while two older boys, Edward and William, did not fall ill. As the Herrs became weaker and sicker, they asked Minerva to take care of the two boys, believing that their own deaths were imminent. According to an observer, Minerva quickly promised the dying mother that she would care for the two youngsters, both of whom were under the age of five. When the police later came to the Herrs' house to burn all of the furnishings in hopes of destroying the yellow fever, they told Minerva to leave town quickly with the children. They explained that officials would forcibly evict her and the children, since the children's parents had died of yellow fever and she had been in the home caring for them. The police might have shown confidence in the Herrs' decision to entrust the care of their children to Minerva, as neither they nor any other townsperson, black or white, stepped forward to care for the two boys. Perhaps fear of contracting yellow fever from young Edward and William stymied any humanitarian efforts on others' parts. Minerva's decision, regardless of the fact that she was the habitual caregiver of the children, shows courage. She took the boys into the woods with her for safety. After the police had completed their efforts to destroy possible sources of contagion at the house, she and the boys clandestinely returned to the home, seeking shelter. The police had left behind some hams and other foodstuffs, so the three were able to live for a while on those provisions.[62]

While hiding in the Herr home, according to documents of the Sisters of Charity, "Minerva took two little sticks of wood and made a little cross out of them. Every morning she would trace a little cross on the boys' breasts and say, 'White chillun, this is all you got to believe in now.'" Neither she nor the boys contracted yellow fever during the epidemic. After the boys spent several months with Minerva, other members of the boys' family, who had sought refuge in the countryside, returned to Holly Springs. Minerva remained with the Herr family until her death. When she died, as a tribute to her devotion and faith, the family gave her "an honorable burial," one with a marker and a fine casket.[63]

Black caregivers were not the only volunteers to provide succor to those afflicted with yellow fever. Rev. Benjamin Black, a black Methodist preacher and former slave, helped both white and black patients in Holly Springs by providing spiritual solace and by keeping an eye on people's property, since law and order was disrupted by the epidemic. As reported in the *Cincinnati Commercial,* Black "has proved invaluable. The colored people who have so heroically stood by us in our hour of peril are represented by this colored minister, of the Methodist Church, who had watched with Christian vigilance the homes of all, without regard to race or previous condition."[64] According to the *Pascagoula Democrat-Star,* Black "at one time [was the] only minister available to console sick and assist at burial" in Holly Springs because of the epidemic's toll. Included in that same report was a poem describing Black's contributions to the relief of the citizens of Holly Springs, both black and white. However, this tribute certainly does not follow the usual flowery testimonials given to whites who aided yellow fever victims and gave spiritual support. Instead, it reveals the racial prejudice existing at the time and diminishes Black's work by using a crude vernacular dialect rather than the more eloquent speech describing those who were white and offering spiritual help.

Only a Nigger Preacher.

He wuz thar when the yeller inflicshun
Come stalkin' 'long over the lan.
An' the hour of awful afflicshun
Show'd us the true grit of er man![65]

A black preacher who helped whites and African Americans alike would probably have been accepted in 1878 southern society because he appeared to be acquiescent to the traditionalists in the town. Nevertheless, at least one home-state newspaper put Rev. Black in his social place by running its "tribute."

Other black ministers also attempted to help fellow African Americans who were affected by the epidemic. In New York City the Colored Preachers' Aid Society sent out a call for help in the *New York Herald:*

To The Colored People of the United States, Especially of the North—
Our people are suffering, dying and destitute. For Heaven's sake relieve
us all you can by sending us means. We are not able to bury our dead or
to nurse and feed the sick and destitute. The most of us have no employment, as all business is suspended. Send us contributions of money or provisions speedily.

    A. Holmes, Chairman Preachers' Aid Society.

    Thomas Shields, Secretary[66]

African Americans in Mississippi were not receiving the aid they needed, whether
from the state, medical groups, or established aid societies.

In Louisiana the situation was different. That state had a longer history of
black benevolent societies, and during the epidemic those entities either picked
up the mantle of charity or reorganized to address the crisis. For example, as discussed by historian Jo Ann Carrigan, black aid societies appeared after the Civil
War in New Orleans, first to address medical and burial needs and later specifically to help groups such as the French-speaking African Americans living in the
city. Societies such as Les Jeunes Amis and La Concorde provided medical assistance to their members. Additionally, unlike Mississippi, New Orleans had black
religious communities like the Sisters of the Holy Family, which offered support
such as nursing care, laundering, and caring for orphans. The Sisters of the Holy
Family tended to both white and black citizens.[67] Mississippi lacked such an
infrastructure, so African Americans had to rely upon the same self-reliance that
their white counterparts were practicing in order to attend to their various needs
throughout the epidemic. Unlike their white counterparts, African Americans
had almost no elite with the power to direct community efforts and resources.

During the epidemic, African Americans did not receive equitable, necessary relief aid. Compounding their tenuous position further, they were often
blamed for transporting yellow fever contagion into other locales. For example,
the second person who died of yellow fever in Jackson was a man who had not
left the city since the imposed quarantine, William McCallum. Local health officials ascertained that McCallum had contracted the disease while visiting the
home of his mother. She lived near Buck Patton, a black man who allegedly allowed his stepson into his home, aware that the young man had come from a
highly infected place. McCallum unknowingly endangered himself simply by
visiting his mother's home. Patton's daughter apparently died of yellow fever a
short time after his stepson arrived. Another African American, Gregg Richards, who lived near Patton, also harbored a quarantine fugitive. Richards died
shortly thereafter. Health officials condemned Patton's and Richards's "criminal
violation[s] of the ordinances which were established to protect the public health"

and pointed out that "unspeakable sorrow" resulted for the McCallum family because of the men's disregard for quarantine lines. No mention was made of Patton's own sorrow at his daughter's death. It is also noteworthy that white people who harbored refugees were not criminalized in this way. Officials soon dispensed disinfectants, which citizens used freely in the neighborhood surrounding the homes of Patton and Richards. Citizens, both white and black, experienced further racial strain as shotgun quarantines tightened around Jackson.[68]

Racial tension was a serious problem when local authorities had to take their own measures, and nowhere was this clearer than in the manning of quarantines. Often, as whites fled to safety, African Americans were the only citizens left in these communities in any significant number, yet whites were hesitant and fearful of recruiting blacks to assist. For example, in early September, Greenville's remaining citizens organized the Greenville Quarantine Guards. The by-laws for the group stated that only white men were qualified to serve. Townsfolk apparently believed that African Americans should not be armed to protect the city, since arming African Americans could aggravate already heightened racial tensions. The Greenville City Council also addressed in a special session the quarantine problems that citizens were attempting to remedy. The resulting ordinance stipulated, "Be it ordained by the Town Council of Greenville, that any person violating any rule or regulation of the Board of Health of said town, or failing to comply with any order of said Board within the time prescribed, shall be deemed guilty of a misdemeanor and upon conviction thereof shall be fined not more than Three Hundred Dollars." The council also appointed a special police militia, with fifty-four members, on August 31 to enforce the city's new law.[69]

With Greenville's citizens well prepared for yellow fever's arrival, how the disease got into the city remains unclear. One report stated that the steamer *City of Vicksburg* imported the contagion on August 14 when she landed two miles above the city. Draymen from the boat and a number of locals interacted. Another possible source was Chinese immigrants on their way to Stoneville, Mississippi, who eluded Greenville's Quarantine Guards. In the early 1870s, planters had recruited Chinese laborers directly from Hong Kong as well as from New Orleans to work on their lands as replacements for African Americans, particularly in Washington County.[70] They reportedly carried the yellow fever contagion with them, as foreigners were suspect. Mysteriously, the Chinese men, according to one account, "by means fair or foul succeeded in having [their] baggage hauled to Greenville and stored for the night in the Engine House, from which place the baggage was transported [the] next day by rail to Stoneville." Contemporaries believed that fomites could hide in baggage and other such items. Lastly, numerous steamboats plying the Mississippi River anchored in Greenville to unload their cargoes and possibly yellow fever contagion, without regard for quarantine restrictions.[71]

Clearly, a good Democratic official was expected to distrust African Americans—although no government solutions to the problem appeared. This paradox of accountability/nonaccountability is evident in a three-page letter that J. H. Campbell of the Grenada City Council addressed to Governor Stone on September 21. Campbell was worried about the situation in Grenada but knew enough not even to ask for help. He explained to the governor his reasons for assuming political control of the city: he was "the only white member of our City-Council left," but a few "Negroes who were members of the council are willing to work with me. I have this day taken charge of city-affairs and appointed a City Marshall & Deputies." Campbell again reported that numerous burglaries had occurred for lack of a law enforcement force. He reiterated that "the Negroes are very insolent, [and] in fact have had charge of the city." Under these desperate circumstances, Campbell (and apparently the black council members) appointed night patrols to guard the city and "to defend ourselves." Surprisingly, the night patrols were "composed of Negroes in whom I have as much confidence as I can place in a negro . . . it is the best I can do." Given the racial situation in 1878 Mississippi, compounded by the fear associated with Grenada's yellow fever epidemic, it is astounding that a white man appointed African Americans to positions of authority. This action reveals desperation on the part of Campbell and the remaining white citizens of Grenada. He qualified his decision, however, by writing that he is "fearful" and "if you could send as many as ten able bodied white men that can be trusted you would be conferring a favor upon the people of our stricken city." Nevertheless, the African-American night patrol was recognized as a necessary means of helping Grenada.[72] Help from the governor was regarded as a favor, not a right—and apparently it never came.

The Grenada African-American guard, though, apparently was not armed, because Campbell asked that white replacements for the black members of the patrol "should be well armed. We in fact have no arms nor can we get them. I have one single barrel derringer and some have nothing." Perhaps his willingness to appoint African Americans to patrol Grenada and its immediate vicinity rested on the fact that they were not armed, nor could they afford weapons. Campbell described the patrol as "poor men and not able to own fire arms." Appointing African Americans to what was in effect militia status, whether armed or unarmed, was certainly an irregularity in race relations in 1878 Mississippi, as African Americans were politically, economically, and socially subordinated. Segregation experienced, if only for a brief time in nineteenth-century Mississippi, moderation.[73]

Campbell wrote a final request to Stone on September 24. From the tone of his letter it is clear that the governor had not sent the requested white, armed replacements to Grenada. Therefore, Campbell demanded "ninety-five stand [sets] of arms and ammunition, [and] a few pistols would be in order. Send me the best guns you can get for my own use and if possible a good pistol as I have only a single barrel derringer." He assured Stone that the munitions "shall be kept in order and only given to responsible parties" and that the city would conduct an election of officers as soon as citizens returned to Grenada. No evidence exists that Campbell ever received arms from the governor.[74]

Further south, officials in Canton complained about that city's black residents, who were probably as unmotivated to help as their white counterparts were—but it was the former who got the blame. The editors of the *American Citizen* lamented that "The negroes here, we are sorry to record it against them, will not work. . . . It is a great favor to get a little washing and ironing done, by paying the most exhorbitant [*sic*] prices." However, in that same issue appears a list of specially appointed policemen that includes the names of three African Americans, Sam Owens, Si Melton, and Ollie Fields. Of the men who had been originally appointed, only four were left by the time the *Citizen* reported this news. That means that only one white man served with the three African Americans to "guard the town and protect the property of those who had fled."[75] The newspaper does not reveal whether or not the men were armed. Nevertheless, the citizens of Canton were indebted to the special lawmen for patrolling the city.

Few instances of relief efforts aimed specifically at African Americans appear in the sources. The state was more concerned with protection against African Americans than with helping them, and local self-help organizations for the most part identified themselves with the Democratic backlash against aid to freedmen. If African Americans wanted help, they too had to help themselves—but with far fewer options. Information regarding an African-American component of and inclusion in aid associations and programs is murky. Newspaper accounts and contemporary observations usually only offered a white perspective of activities geared at relieving those burdened with financial problems created by the yellow fever epidemic. However, the *New York Herald* reported that in Washington, D.C., African Americans raised $123 in early September through church collections and individual contributions. Nevertheless, no specific donors' names, church affiliations, or indications of the money's destination appear, although news accounts often printed such information describing white relief efforts. Any mention of black participation in and receipt of relief aid was refracted only through white reports.[76]

Despite the ill treatment afforded them in relief disbursement, African Americans contributed money and supplies to relief efforts. Especially notable is a donation from Macon, Mississippi. On September 9, George G. Dillard, Macon's mayor, reported to J. L. Power that "The colored people here . . . raised fifty-one dollars and sent it to Grenada. The ladies . . . [sent] sheets, towels, pillow cases, etc., if such things . . . [were] needed." He also asked if Grenada could use some live poultry from the "colored folk," who "can get up a large quantity."[77] Dillard must have met with the African-American community in Macon to collect the monetary and material donations. The actions of African Americans in Macon probably exemplify other such efforts throughout Mississippi during the 1878 epidemic. However, those gestures will more than likely remain unknown, because during this time in Mississippi the black community lacked the means to document its participation in relief efforts.

In spite of problems for African Americans centering on relief distribution, other efforts to provide aid to their communities occurred. The black population of Port Gibson elected a representative to organize relief efforts there. Thomas Richardson was the president of the black counterpart of the white Port Gibson Howard Association.[78] Presumably, he was the liaison between the two groups, so in this case communication and coordination between whites and African Americans probably occurred.

During the 1878 yellow fever epidemic, the color line occasionally frayed as extraordinary circumstances created windows of opportunity for African Americans to participate in charitable and relief efforts, both within their own communities and in those of whites. However, these anomalies existed only briefly, as Mississippi society and politicians buttressed the infrastructure for Jim Crowism even before the 1890 state constitution.[79] As so often in Mississippi history, racial tension kept interest away from much more burning social needs—in this case, care of the victims of yellow fever.

5
The Human Suffering

The cup of sorrow had been drained to the dregs.
—*Cincinnati Commercial*, September 17, 1878

Mississippians' suffering was appalling. It is clear that the absence of a health plan by the state exacerbated an already critical situation. Therefore, it is instructive to consider the human suffering during the yellow fever epidemic with a consideration of what might have been done and what grassroots efforts and infrastructures were created during the epidemic to distribute money and provisions.

A first case study is Vicksburg. By September 7 the town had recorded 2,500 cases of yellow fever as the populace began its descent into a full-blown epidemic. This number is staggering. Vicksburg had a pre-1878 population of 14,000, but 6,000 had fled from yellow fever, so nearly a third of the people left in town had fallen ill. This city had been the first to be affected by yellow fever in late July and early August, so city officials had established quarantine lines earlier than officials in other towns had. By September, however, Vicksburg was a city in mourning. The Frank J. Fisher Funeral Home was one of the most lucrative businesses in Vicksburg during this month. The quarantine hindered all other commerce severely. In two accounting volumes, the proprietors of the funeral home recorded the daily procedures and costs of each funeral. For example, Willie Spengler, one of the three sons of the Spengler family that eventually purchased Cooper's Well, died of yellow fever on September 3. The entry states that he was "21 yrs. 4 mos." and was buried in "One plain box." The Spengler family hired a hearse from the funeral home and also paid for a burial robe—both extravagances for a funeral at this time. The total cost for Willie's funeral was $112, definitely one of the more expensive arrangements in plague-ridden and quarantined Vicksburg. Often, families of yellow fever victims could not even afford caskets for their loved ones. The Howard Association, as one aspect of their benevolent work, would then pay for the service and necessary funeral items. On September 12 the benevolent group paid the funeral home nine dollars for three simple coffins. Many entries in that business's accounts illustrate the Howards' generosity.[1]

Moreover, the relief aid provided by the Howards reflects economic hardship among Vicksburg's remaining citizens. At the beginning of September, few entries in the funeral home's records recognize the Howards' beneficence, indicating that most citizens were able to pay funeral expenses. By the end of the month, however, the majority of the entries are for five-dollar Howard funerals. The Howards, in turn, relied upon donations nationwide to accomplish their work. This pattern in Vicksburg illustrates that deprivations from the quarantine restrictions created economic difficulties for the city's populace, leaving many without the resources to pay funeral costs. After two months of quarantine, stagnation set in for the city's businesses. Vicksburg's citizens were overwhelmed with yellow fever and had no resources left, not even those needed to pay for family members' and friends' funerals. Despite this hardship, the city's officials still maintained the quarantine lines—a self-imposed siege.[2]

The state government was unable to offer aid to Vicksburg, as it was also struggling to recover from years of Reconstruction and economic hard times. With the largest number of yellow fever cases compared to other infected cities in the state, Vicksburg battled to maintain itself economically, also. The populace would have to care for themselves with the help of outside resources.

In September, yellow fever also overwhelmed Greenville, another major town on the Mississippi, about seventy-five miles north of Vicksburg, with 144 cases and 41 deaths. Before the epidemic, 2,800 people had lived there. As with other Mississippi municipalities, panic ensued once news of Yellow Jack filtered into the area, and only about 1,300 people remained in the city when the dust cleared. Before the quarantine commenced, the Greenville, Columbus, and Birmingham Railroad advertised a free run to Stoneville, nine miles east, for Greenville's citizens. People believed Stoneville to be a safe locale, as it was outside Greenville's city limits. The attorneys for the rail line, Percy and Yeager, advertised that the August 31 evening train would be the last run out of Greenville. The trip would be free for all those who desired to leave, and Greenville's citizens could bring "household effects." These complimentary rides and freight-hauling trips demonstrate another example of the outpouring of assistance to the state. Rev. Stevenson Archer, the local Presbyterian minister, recounted to J. L. Power that "a fearful havoc [had] been made among the citizens of our beautiful little town," and only a portion of the people remained "to face the grim destroyer."[3] Many inhabitants of the town took advantage of the free transportation provided by the Greenville, Columbus, and Birmingham Railroad to avoid becoming isolated in Greenville. Like other towns along the river and railroad lines, Greenville faced the loss of key personnel and the majority of the town's citizens; therefore, problems in commerce, civic organization, and law enforcement resulted.

Even disposal of the dead was regulated only at the local level, breeding fear even if rotting corpses did not breed the disease. Many cemeteries across the state filled to capacity during September. The small town of Lake, located in Scott County on the Vicksburg and Meridian Railroad line, had a population of about 350 in 1878. When the town's officials received the yellow fever news in late August, they declared an immediate quarantine and created a Citizens' Aid Association. However, the Sneed family from Vicksburg entered the town with special permission as they sought refuge early in September. Mrs. Sneed was the daughter of Colonel J. S. Yarborough, Lake's mayor, so officials allowed the couple in. Such decisions were local, and officials catered to the wishes of local elites. Mr. Sneed soon developed what local health officials labeled as a "slight malarial attack," since city bureaucrats did not want to admit to having made a mistake by allowing him to break the quarantine lines. Sneed's brother-in-law, Lee Scott, accommodated the Sneeds at his home, where he could oversee proper nursing care. Kittie Scott, Lee's wife and Sneed's sister, helped tend to Sneed while he was in the Scotts' home. Additionally, during Sneed's convalescence, a group of five friends gathered daily in his room to play chess and various card games. Sneed's servant, George Jones, an African American, was also continuously in the sickroom. Within two weeks after Sneed's arrival in Lake, all of his friends and his servant had died of yellow fever, as did Mayor Yarborough. Kittie and Lee Scott also died. Sneed himself recovered.[4]

By September 22, twenty more deaths in Lake had resulted from yellow fever. Dr. George C. McCallum and his wife, Mary, both died during this time, as did their two young daughters, May and Kate. Officials hurriedly buried the bodies of the victims in Lake Cemetery, about a half mile from town. However, on the night of September 22 a tremendous rainstorm arrived and pounded the area for almost two days, washing out the shallow, newly dug graves and exposing the corpses. After the storm, caretakers refilled the graves and spread carbolic acid and lime over the area to disinfect it. Many Mississippians believed that miasma from rotting corpses could cause yellow fever and thus hurried these reburials in Lake Cemetery. Firmer guidelines about how to bury victims of yellow fever, even if unsupported by state inspections, would have helped in this instance. In fact, the Pass Christian City Council passed an ordinance that levied a ten-dollar fine for digging up any yellow fever victim "in less than 18 months after death," so great was the fear of contagion from corpses.[5] Unfortunately, the efforts in Lake were useless; by the end of September, health officials had recorded approximately 330 cases of yellow fever in and around the city.[6]

Approximately 170 miles north of Lake, Grenada had a population of approximately 2,500 preceding the epidemic, of whom about 1,300 were white and 1,200 were African American or of mixed race. One report stated that "after the stampede" out of town to flee the yellow plague, only 325 whites and about

1,000 African Americans remained in the town. A Mrs. Fields, who contracted the first case of yellow fever in Grenada, died at the end of July. Her physicians labeled her death malarial congestive fever, but she had exhibited the characteristic black vomit and yellow skin. Local health officials did not want to admit that yellow fever was in Grenada.[7]

From the time of Mrs. Fields's death until the end of August, trains continued to operate between Memphis and Grenada. In September, officials in Grenada established quarantines around the city, but railroad traffic continued. Trains were ordered to pass through town at about fifty miles per hour, as officials believed that such a speed could prevent the yellow fever contagion from escaping the cars. C. S. Spinzig stated that the trains crossed "the bridge over the Yalabusha [sic] River at such velocity that human life was most frivolously exposed to the danger of the breaking of those usually frail structures."[8] State authorities should have taken a leading role in halting the running of unnecessary trains, setting clear rules for interaction, and making sure that trains did convey necessary foodstuffs. Passengers between the two junctions disembarked outside the city limits and then made their way into Grenada, often bypassing quarantine lines. Grenada's yellow fever contagion undoubtedly originated from Memphis, which experienced its own yellow fever epidemic. The railroad cars were ideal transporters for *Aedes aegypti* mosquitoes and persons harboring the virus.

Impoverished Mississippi was a good breeding ground for disease, and local officials often hit on the true underlying cause of the disease, even though they blamed it on smells rather than mosquitoes. For instance, local health officials in Grenada attempted to trace the origin of the contagion to that city's grossly neglected sanitary situation. Privy vaults or outhouses had been used for years with no cleaning, people's backyards were neglected, and "hog wallows" abounded within the town; furthermore, a drainage culvert ran diagonally across the town and emptied into the Yalobusha River. Regardless of the origin of contagion, by September the "yellow peril" confronted Grenada's remaining citizens. There were 690 reported cases with 274 deaths by the end of the month. As J. L. Power recorded, "The plague destroyed social organization and the mechanism of civilization as if they had been living beings. Law and police, the board of health and the relief committee, were all stopped by death." The *Pascagoula Democrat-Star* lamented that Grenada was "no longer a city," it was "a morgue."[9] Again, the situation in Grenada provided a good example of local governmental failure in providing assistance to its citizens and demonstrated the need for outside help. State officials were clearly unwilling to call on United States soldiers for help in maintaining law and order, although that resource existed.

A series of telegrams to Governor Stone from D. W. Coan, Grenada's Howard Association manager, and J. H. Campbell, a citizen of the town, illustrates the dire circumstances in Grenada and reveals the disgruntlement with the failure of state authorities to fix problems resulting from yellow fever. On September 18, Coan telegraphed Stone explaining that "Some of the colored people in subordination [sic]. One man has already stabbed his wife and no place to put him and no authorities here now living. What shall we do with the man under arrest. I am alone guarding the town." Coan wrote Stone later that same day that C. T. Jackson, who was supposedly organizing relief efforts for Grenada, had been accused of stealing yellow fever victims' watches and money. Apparently, the evidence was convincing, for he had been arrested. Coan again asked, "What shall I do?" He closed the communiqué with "Answer." Coan was impatient because of the stressful environment and Stone's lack of response. He explained in his final telegram that "There is no sheriff nor any other officer county or city not even an alderman. Cannot you deputise [sic] some one as sheriff. Something must be done[.] Answer."[10] There is no record of any answer.

On September 21, J. H. Campbell, a member of the Grenada City Council, assumed control of the city's civic affairs. Presumably, Campbell believed it was his duty as an elected official and leading citizen to wrest control from unscrupulous persons in Grenada who were taking advantage of a horrible situation. Despite Campbell's best efforts at maintaining law and order and guarding quarantine lines, 274 yellow fever deaths occurred by the end of September in Grenada, along with an undetermined amount of larceny and property destruction. An especially distressing scenario in the city involved the Fields family. Mrs. Fields went to the train station to make plans for her daughter's evacuation, and health officials believed she was infected there. She died shortly thereafter. At her funeral, several family members and friends described a terrible smell. A crack in Mrs. Field's casket caused a stench so overwhelming that a "great nausea" overcame many who were nearby. Some contemporary accounts blamed this leak as the source of yellow fever contagion, since so many of the people attending the funeral later died. For example, out of thirteen members of Mrs. Field's family at the funeral, ten had yellow fever by the end of September. Only three recovered. In this instance, a mother, two sons, a daughter, and grandchildren all died of yellow fever. This wholesale destruction of families in Mississippi was not an unusual occurrence.[11] A contemporary commented that nothing could illustrate the severity of the disease except to explain "that during its prevalence there was only a single death from any other cause than the yellow fever." The president of the Grenada County Board of Health reported to the state board of health that Grenada had approximately 1,050 yellow fever cases. Out of that number, roughly 350 died.

The death ratio of white to black in Grenada was very disproportionate. Of the approximate 350 deaths, 260 were whites and 90 were African Americans.

An eyewitness noted that even though many African Americans in Grenada went to the countryside refugee camps to escape yellow fever, most returned before the pestilence ended. The majority of the citizens in Grenada during the epidemic's course were African American, as illustrated by J. H. Campbell's integration action to create a protective city militia. The observer further stated that "as a rule, the Negroes took the disease later in the season than the whites," and "the disease among them was of a much milder character than the whites."[12] As a result, many contemporaries erroneously believed that African Americans were immune to yellow fever. Records listing case and fatality numbers did indicate that African Americans fared better in combating the disease and apparently did have a resistance to yellow fever. Recent studies have found that "ninety percent or more of black cases [of yellow fever] survived."[13] According to 1878 records, only four white people in Grenada did not contract the fever.[14] Such disproportionate suffering must have left white Mississippians feeling ever more strongly that their world was askew.

Port Gibson's tribulations mirrored those of Grenada in September 1878. John Kelly reported in the *Port Gibson Reveille* that during the epidemic he and his family had gone to the home of Mrs. Mackey, about three miles from town. After the Kellys arrived, it was not long before yellow fever came to visit, too. "Everybody in the house, even the Negroes, had the fever except me," Kelly recalled. "There were no nurses so I had to wait on the sick. I . . . got the wood and hauled the water from the spring, went to town, as far as the quarantine station, for everything they needed and did not take the fever." Neither Kelly nor Mackey contracted yellow fever, even though they were in the midst of a "pest house."[15]

The Shreves, another Port Gibson family, experienced three deaths in September. Charles Shreve, his wife, and their son Charles Jr. all died within eleven days of one another. A newspaper obituary reported that "the horrors of the epidemic were most fully displayed in the sufferings of this family. Three out of four of those who remained at home and were exposed to the disease were swept away. No higher rate of mortality was suffered by any family in our plague-stricken community." The Pearsons, too, lost a son to yellow fever. Written in the Pearson family Bible is this entry: "Henry Hume—Born at Rose Cottage, April 19, 1856 8:00 a.m." Directly below his birth announcement, his death entry simply states, "At Grand Gulf Miss. 1:30 a.m. Henry Hume Pearson Sept 13th 1878 Aged 22." Both of these Port Gibson families lost sons who were "plucked in the flower of their youth."[16]

During September, commerce in Port Gibson and general downtown activity halted as a result of the fever. Silence reigned. When outside help finally arrived, physicians and nurses discovered that practically every home was a hospital. The nurses did their best, but the yellow fever did not abate. "Corpses, just as the victims died, wrapped in sheets and blankets, and hurriedly encoffined, were stealthily lifted out of doors and sometimes out of windows, and buried in haste at sunrise, after dark by dim lanterns, and frequently lay all night long in the graveyard, unburied," recounted Dr. J. P. Dromgoole. Quick, secretive burials were commonplace as families did not want to call attention to the fact that yellow fever was among them and possibly risk social ostracism. One poor mother who could locate no assistance dug her own baby's grave after the child died of yellow fever. By September 10 health officials had recorded 475 yellow fever cases and 85 deaths; on September 23, reports indicated 600 cases and 104 deaths.[17]

Vicksburg's populace also struggled during September. After Paul Stoltz's death in July, the town's citizens endured extreme hardships as the epidemic spread and intensified. By September 6 officials reported 1,395 cases and 309 deaths. As the *New York Herald* reported, "the whizz of the wheels on the doctors' carriages as they drive at full speed indicates an increase too surely." Another witness reported to J. L. Power that the "suffering from the pestilence [was] fearful . . . we have seen the horrors of the battlefield, and have tasted the sorrows and deprivations of prison life, have buried comrades and friends on lonely, far-off battlefields, but we have never, in a varied and eventful life, witnessed anything which so awakened the sensibilities of our nature." By the end of September, health officials listed 4,226 cases of yellow fever and 849 resultant deaths.[18]

Greenville's remaining populace also experienced a horrific September. The town's paper was reduced from four pages to two because quarantines blocked outside news sources. Still, Power reported that on a single day, September 18, twenty-four people had died. Reporters described the day as a "black" one for the citizens of Greenville. The overwhelming number of victims in such a brief period resulted in a critical shortage of coffins, and John Manifold, Greenville's undertaker, had also died on that dreadful day. To deal with the growing numbers of dead, some local citizens organized themselves into a burial committee. According to one account, "there was not a casket left, so they commandeered lumber and men and made plain, unpainted wooden boxes, which served for rich and poor, white and black alike. No longer could the question of family plot in the cemetery be considered. Instead, there were mass graves dug in long rows, to stand in readiness as the victims fell."[19]

It was also well within the state government's ability to take actions to cause cash flow during the crisis. Greenville's citizens were also hard-pressed for cash during September, since the epidemic interrupted financial activities on all levels. Bank officers in Greenville had locked citizens' savings in the local bank's vault, but by the end of September the bank personnel were all dead from yellow fever, leaving no one who knew the combination to the vault. Therefore, officials in

Vicksburg sent a steamboat upriver to bring currency to Greenville's citizens so they could purchase much-needed supplies from local merchants. Under normal circumstances, Mississippi's citizens, especially farmers, relied upon store credit to purchase their necessary items. Historian Ted Ownby asserts that by 1890, southerners were on the verge of a "change in the history of consumer behavior" as a result of mass production and distribution, expanding railroad systems, and ready cash resulting from greater employment opportunities, including those for women. However, during the yellow fever epidemic, store owners demanded cash for goods because they feared that the customer would not live long enough to pay off a debt. In Greenville, no one could access the bank's assets, so citizens had no way to purchase goods.[20] In the absence of help from the state government, local initiative guaranteed the citizens of Greenville some relief.

Greenville's health officials adhered to the state board of health's recommended methods of disinfecting their town, attempted to manage its burgeoning yellow fever situation, and soothed the remaining residents' growing fears. Despite earnest efforts, the city's officials were unable to maintain health standards, and by early September the number of yellow fever cases had mushroomed to 250, with 151 deaths. Citizens had tried to halt the proliferation of the disease by disinfecting throughout late August, but to no avail. It was reported in the *Greenville Times* that "lime filled the drains and ditches, [and] crude carbolic acid was scattered in every direction and filled the air with its offensive odors while the black cloud of burning sulphur brought vividly to mind Dante's description of the inferno." Following the state board's recommendation, the clothing and bedding of the dead were burned to eradicate all yellow fever fomites. Moreover, some citizens actually hung carcasses of raw beef around their homes to ward off the yellow fever. The rationale behind this gruesome spectacle remains unknown.[21] Perhaps it was believed that the rotting meat would attract any contagion floating through the air.

The response of Greenville's citizens was typical. About two hundred citizens convened at the council room to assess the shotgun quarantine around the city and to establish further health regulations. As this mass town meeting attests, the democratic process had not completely broken down in Greenville during the epidemic. However, the meeting was only for white men. They were on the second-story gallery of the building when their combined weight proved to be too much for the structure to support. The building's second floor collapsed, and four of the men suffered broken legs. The *Pascagoula Democrat-Star* printed a report of the accident and stated that "since yellow fever was declared epidemic in Greenville . . . 40 deaths have occurred, while 125 cases remain under treatment."[22] Lists of yellow fever victims appeared in the newspaper along with relief contributions and offers of assistance.

Four plantation owners who lived south of Greenville placed the following notice in the city's newspaper: "We the Planters, residents of places below Greenville on Rattlesnake Bayou and river roads . . . Do hereby resolve that we hold ourselves in readiness to forward such supplies in [the] shape of poultry and provisions. . . . Any request made by the Mayor or other proper authority, will be promptly met."[23] J. R. Shields, Jasper Archer Jr., T. B. Warfield, and Carnal Warfield signed the proposal.

Outside aid continued to flow into the city also. The New York City Chamber of Commerce sent $1,500 to Greenville's stricken citizens, and doctors from other locales came to help. Dr. W. B. Archer of Point Coupee, Louisiana, arrived in Greenville believing he was immune to yellow fever because he had survived the disease when he was a child. He had underestimated the virulence of this contagion, however, and soon appeared on the death rolls. By September 14 three more doctors were ill, leaving the city almost bereft of medical aid. Still, the disease did not abate, and regardless of these relief efforts, the citizens of Greenville suffered greatly. The *New Orleans Picayune* quoted the captain of the *Ben Allen,* a steamer still operating in the Greenville area: "Situation is horrible [in Greenville]. 400 remain and cannot get away; 200 sick; nearly 100 deaths. No boats running; telegraph line down for about ten days; cannot make their wants known; are shut out from the world. For God's sake get nurses, supplies, and money on other boats."[24]

By September 27, health officers reported 227 yellow fever deaths in Greenville. According to Power, the names of the victims filled two and a half columns in the next day's *Greenville Times.* At the end of the month, twenty-six more people in the city had died, including Mayor A. B. Trigg, three councilmen, and the city's marshal, attorney, assessor, and street supervisor.[25] It appears that these men had remained behind to maintain some local governmental control, performing organizational and regulatory duties. This scenario played out in many other communities, resulting in the loss of nearly all local officials.

Because quarantine efforts did little to stem the spread of yellow fever in September, citizens along the Mississippi Gulf Coast continued to cope with the disease during that month. On September 13 the *Pascagoula Democrat-Star* reported numerous cases and deaths in several coastal cities. Bay St. Louis had reported twenty-five yellow fever cases and five deaths, and the New Orleans Howard Association had sent four nurses and one physician to Bay St. Louis to help with the mounting yellow fever cases. Pass Christian had reported sixteen cases and two deaths by the same date. The fever was spreading throughout the coastal communities in Hancock, Harrison, and Jackson counties.[26]

Pass Christian, a small "watering place" and post village in western Harrison County, some fifty-seven miles from New Orleans, also experienced distress as yellow fever appeared within its boundaries. The village had a population of 1,250 before the epidemic. Unlike other Mississippi towns, however, its population did not decrease because of yellow fever panic; it more than doubled. Hordes of refugees from New Orleans flocked to the "Pass" seeking safety from Bronze John. On September 1, physicians listed only two cases of yellow fever near Pass Christian's steamboat wharf, but by September 10 officials confirmed ten to fifteen cases in the same neighborhood, the point at which New Orleans refugees landed. Pass Christian's officials were not prepared for the influx of refugees, and only one doctor, George N. Smith, treated the majority of yellow fever cases in the village.[27]

Other coastal locations recorded mounting yellow fever cases and deaths through the month. By September 27, Logtown, a small village in Hancock County on the Pearl River, listed 19 cases of fever among its 400 inhabitants. The yellow fever at Logtown was particularly virulent. The first case was Edward Christian, an African American from New Orleans. according to records, Christian received good care and recovered. Robert Carrie was the first official yellow fever death in the community. As one observer noted, Carrie was "honored and loved by the whole community." Another victim, Kimball Roberts, was "one of the most promising young men on Pearl River." A heartbroken mother mourned the death of her three sons when Forrest, William, and Tom Leonard died from the "yellow plague."[28]

Further east along the coast, the town of Handsboro had a population of about four hundred prior to the epidemic. As with most other coastal villages, Handsboro's first case of fever was a New Orleanian, George Jeremyn, who was fleeing that city's epidemic. Jeremyn arrived on a schooner from New Orleans and displayed yellow fever symptoms on September 2. His attending physician, Dr. John E. Lyon, was a native of Georgia and had married Emma H. Liddle on September 1, only a day before the infection appeared. More than likely, as a result of his marriage to a local woman, Lyon planned to remain in the Handsboro area in spite of the yellow fever threat; therefore, he treated Jeremyn the day after his marriage.[29]

By September 13, Jeremyn was recuperating under Lyon's care; others, however, were not as fortunate. Mateo Poleicho, a native of Dalmatia in the Austrian Empire, lived in Handsboro and fished for his livelihood. He had recently become engaged to a young Nickols girl, and the two sought refuge at John Latimer's home, two miles north of Handsboro. While with the Latimer family, Poleicho fell ill, and Dr. Lyon traveled to examine him. Lyon pronounced the sickness yellow fever. Upon hearing that news, Latimer and his family packed a few belongings and fled into the countryside. Poleicho's fiancée remained with her "intended," and "with the devotion characteristic of the sex, nursed and attended to the wants of the doomed man, who died next day." Her father, Jack Nickols, then arranged for Poleicho's burial just a few feet from the house in which he died.[30]

Mississippians gratefully accepted provisions and financial aid from outside sources during September as they dealt with dire situations. According to contemporary accounts, monetary contributions from sundry locales and organizations throughout the United States, including American residents in Mexico City and even Secretary of State William H. Evarts, flowed to Mississippians. These funds "did much to alleviate the privations and suffering of those who were rendered helpless through the ravages of the pestilence." Appeals for aid appeared in newspapers across the country. The *Cincinnati Star* best summarized the national opinion: "Therefore let no man . . . withhold his cash sympathies from the plague-stricken people of the South. The fear of misappropriation should furnish no excuse for delay . . . the cash and supplies forwarded for the relief of the Southern people pass through the hands of those who at the risk of their own lives have stood by their dying neighbors. Such people can be trusted with untold treasures." The *Detroit Free Press* solicited funds specifically for the city of Jackson and received $50. On September 28, several organizations in California, including St. John's Episcopal Church in San Francisco and Wells, Fargo and Company, sent $2,254 to Governor Stone for distribution among the yellow fever victims in the state.[31] Donations sent specifically to the governor's office were pooled with the Masons' monies and allocated to citizens throughout the state. Approximately $7,000 was sent to Stone throughout the epidemic.[32] Money poured into the state from individuals, also. For example, E. P. Jacobson of Denver, Colorado, sent $100 for relief measures. Philanthropists repeated these gestures of goodwill throughout September and beyond, eventually contributing the impressive sum of $522,632.42, with an additional $1,675 coming from foreign sources.[33]

Often, local health officials allotted monies directly to the stricken families, while at other times the donations augmented cities' coffers for relief committees. For example, on September 27, the family of Rev. John McCampbell in Grenada received $150 to help defray their expenses after McCampbell's death from yellow fever. Simultaneously, the Grenada Howard Association Office received $1,000 for its humanitarian efforts in that city. An attempt appears to have been made to distribute funds equitably, but more tended to go to distressed white families.[34]

Monetary aid to Mississippians, however, was not limited to sources outside the state. Many Mississippians contributed to the relief efforts of their neighbors. Fellow Mississippians generously supported their stricken brothers and sisters in 1878 by devising distinctive fund-raising activities. By September 30, citizens from Baldwyn, Houston, Kosciusko, Liberty, Scranton, State Line, and Terry had collected $4,862.36 for their fellow citizens. Governor Stone even donated $100 to the people of the state.[35]

The majority of Mississippians considered it the "duty of our citizens in healthy localities to contribute . . . to the relief of the sick and suffering."[36] Citizens in Mississippi raised funds for assistance efforts in a variety of ways to help others in the state cope with yellow fever and its accompanying quarantine restrictions. People in Biloxi organized an entertainment at Oak Cottage and charged a 25¢ admission fee. This event grossed $300—either twelve hundred people attended this entertainment or some gave larger donations to the cause. Whichever was the case, events such as these provided significant amounts of money for suffering Mississippians. On September 6 in Pascagoula, young ladies and gentlemen of the Pascagoula Amateur Dramatics Club gave an entertainment at Scranton Academy for the benefit and relief of yellow fever victims in Vicksburg and Port Gibson. Locals from Scranton, Moss Point, and Seashore attended this event. Fund-raisers such as these were indicative of grassroots-level efforts throughout the state where local talent participated. At Scranton Academy, a banjo solo by Mr. McCullum and "jigs" by Messrs. Davidson and Lyons were part of the entertainment, as was an oratorical "Sermon" in which Mr. W. A. Henslee parodied an African-American preacher. Presumably, African Americans did not participate in this event. Amanda Krebs also donated a piece of needlework to be raffled. Advertisements billed this show as a "charitable and commendable undertaking" with delicious refreshments provided by the women. Local homemakers donated ten cakes for the refreshments. Admission was 50¢ for gentlemen and 25¢ for women and children. The entertainment earned $127.44 for yellow fever victims in Vicksburg and Port Gibson.[37]

Perhaps the most important way in which state officials could have helped to relieve suffering would have been to provide an administrative structure to coordinate charitable distributions to the needy. But the charitable organizations had to take on that role, too. To disburse funds raised through local events such as those in Pascagoula, Howards often organized relief efforts. Howards from other locales, such as New Orleans or Memphis, often had to manage relief efforts outside their immediate jurisdiction, because some communities simply did not have the required personnel remaining in the environs. They had either fled or died in the epidemic; consequently, Howards from other cities faced the daunting challenge of not only sustaining Mississippians with relief aid but also creating the infrastructure to distribute provisions and financial assistance. In most infected areas, officials attempted to create their own Howard associations so that they could alleviate yellow fever problems on a local level. However, that was not always possible because of the vagaries of the yellow fever epidemic.

If no local Howard Association existed or could be created, outside Howards responded quickly to appeals for aid. Regardless of origination point, Howards were an integral element in relief efforts for Mississippi.

Grenada asked the Howards for additional medical personnel to fill the vacuum created by the yellow fever epidemic in that town. By September, the city's doctors and nurses had either died or were so exhausted that Grenada had virtually no medical coverage. Officials telegraphed Howards in various locations, begging for twenty-five nurses to come and tend yellow fever victims. The city's officials even offered the exorbitant salary of five dollars per day if a nurse answered their plea. One young telegraph worker, who had continued to send appeals and news reports from Grenada, alerted the outside world and Howard associations to Grenada's plight as the plague reached its zenith in September. Through the hot September days, the adolescent telegraph operator stayed at his post, ever tapping out entreaties for help and descriptions of horror. According to Dr. John Brownrigg of Columbus, Mississippi, "Corpses rotted in the sun on the platform at the depot, but the boy operator stifled the odor with a handkerchief soaked in carbolic acid solution and kept his finger on the instrument [telegraph]. . . . The boy operator moved the heart of Christendom with his simple words, describing the sufferings of the people, and succor came at last." The Howard Association sent personnel and aid and revived hope "in the hearts of the stricken people. . . . Helpless women and children, trembling in the agony of despair, cling to them as their deliverers."[38] This unnamed youth rose to the challenge, but the government officials should have done the job.

In response to Grenada's requests for help, the Memphis Howards sent Colonel Butler P. Anderson and General William J. Smith to organize relief efforts and aid distribution. As in so many cases, the leaders were former Confederate officers. According to contemporary accounts, Anderson and Smith "worked and toiled day and night unflinchingly." Unfortunately, Anderson died in Grenada while unselfishly helping others. The New Orleans Howards also sent two physicians, Drs. Mandeville and H. A. Veazie, and sixteen nurses to Grenada to assist that city's fever-stricken citizens and one remaining doctor, H. J. Ray, president of the Grenada County Board of Health. Additionally, Dr. Woolfolk of Kentucky volunteered his professional services to Grenada. Sadly, he soon appeared on the city's death roll. Those citizens remaining in the city received additional money and provisions from the Howards and outside sources. Contributions to Grenada totaled $19,818, while disbursements equaled $20,240, an impressive amount that could have provided help to all citizens in Grenada, black and white. Grenada had done well, thanks to private initiative, but the resources of a state government, even in 1878 Mississippi, could have reached out to a much wider audience and channeled donations to where they were most needed.

Relief efforts in Grenada continued throughout September, and statistics reveal that yellow fever had begun to wane by the end of the month. After running its course through the urban population, the disease began working its way out into the countryside. According to popular assumptions at that time, the reason for this spread was that no more potential victims were left in the city. "For want of material" became the catchphrase in reports throughout the state, especially in towns that had experienced the height of the epidemic in September. From Grenada came this news on October 1: "The terrible fever scourge having run its course at this place, there is no further need of money or supplies. Our people can never forget the open-handed generosity with which their wants have been supplied by North, South, East and West alike."[39]

Such a statement again drives home the lesson that whether Mississippi liked it or not, the state was indeed part of a larger country. And, when it came to help with yellow fever, Mississippians had the grace to be grateful. Recent scholarship has even suggested that as a result of the outpouring of support to Mississippians and other southerners during the 1878 epidemic, Mississippians "reconceptualized" northerners and all others who just thirteen years earlier had been potential enemies in the Civil War. As Edward J. Blum explains, "The epidemic allowed them [southerners] a moment to surrender symbolically to the nation without acknowledging any past wrong or guilt." In essence, the South was not "defeated during the Civil War or because of slavery," but by disease and northern generosity. The horror of the 1878 yellow fever epidemic overshadowed once-fierce sectional antagonism.[40]

Major urban centers in the state best exemplify Mississippians' dependence upon outside assistance during the epidemic. For example, Vicksburg appealed to outside sources for help during September, as its yellow fever case and death numbers increased. Vicksburg's mayor, the secretary of the local Howard Association, the county treasurer, and the telegraph operator all died from the pestilence during September. Eight physicians were working nonstop during that time to help the victims of the scourge, but they could not meet the continuous demand for assistance. Therefore, officials issued an appeal for additional medical personnel. Since yellow fever had established itself in Vicksburg, the disease had raged unchecked; the city was desperate for medicines, nurses, and foodstuffs to aid its suffering citizens. About thirty doctors answered the Howards' call to help the citizens of Vicksburg. Of these volunteers, nine died. Dr. A. R. Green, an African American who volunteered his medical expertise, died of the scourge in Vicksburg. Powers stated that he "did good work for many days" but was eventually "numbered with the dead." Two local physicians also died in September along with the volunteers. One account states that the two "were armed alone with undaunted courage and faith in the power of medicine" yet "fell with their harness [faith], trying to relieve their suffering race, and to establish that the science of physic is mighty, and must prevail over disease." All of these physicians, local and volunteer, died while "battling at the front to save the stricken and doomed, or standing valiantly at the posts to which they were assigned by duty, unswerved by the dreadful devastation surrounding them."[41]

In September some cities in Mississippi were finally able to organize their own Howard associations. On September 10 the citizens of Handsboro created their Howard branch. Ironically, the purpose of this association, as reported in the *Pascagoula Democrat-Star,* was initially "to procure money and delicacies" for yellow fever victims in New Orleans. No mention appeared regarding the needs of the local citizens.[42] Whatever the intent, Handsboro officials were still able to organize a relief association. To cope with the overwhelming demand for food and medical supplies during September, the citizens of Port Gibson also organized a local Howard Association. Members elected Jas. A. Gage as president and Horace Smith Fulkerson as the secretary and treasurer. The town had very few healthy people, but these two men did their best and tried to distribute equitably the relief materials, including coffins.[43]

Yellow fever caused an altered state of existence in Mississippi during the epidemic of 1878. The lives of Mississippians were transformed irrevocably because of a chance encounter with an *A. aegypti* mosquito carrying the yellow fever virus. As a reporter from the *Pascagoula Democrat-Star* observed, "Whenever you see two or three of our citizens talking on the street you may bet your bottom dollar they are discussing either the quarantine or yellow fever subject." Some towns in the state had a brief experience with the disease while their sister communities suffered greatly. For example, Iuka, located in the northeast corner of state on the Memphis and Charlestown Railroad, had only six yellow fever cases and three deaths out of a population of about a thousand. Iuka was the hometown of Governor Stone but was not a likely place for refugees. Compared to other locales in the state, these numbers are astonishing, particularly since Iuka established no quarantine restrictions. Yellow fever also lightly affected other communities across Mississippi. On September 20, E. Merrill, a local official of Iuka, informed Stone that "Few cases bilious fever here all getting well. No yellow fever whatever. People all well. Town as healthy as this time last year."[44]

Likewise, Natchez miraculously escaped yellow fever contagion in the 1878 epidemic, even though it had been affected by the 1853 epidemic and was located on the Mississippi River. City officials had established a rigid quarantine around its boundaries and along the Mississippi early in the epidemic, and Natchez recorded no yellow fever deaths during this outbreak. In fact, it is the one location where quarantine regulations appear to have been effective. It is difficult, however, to know if it was the quarantine or some other unknown factor that kept Natchez fever-free.

Because the epidemic interrupted commerce and communication throughout the state, even those Mississippi towns not directly affected by the disease suffered. Fear permeated all communities in the state. Religious activities fell by the wayside, and education came to a standstill. Because of the quarantine restrictions, few outside business transactions were conducted in most Mississippi towns. Cotton remained unpicked where yellow fever raged through the autumn months because no workers were available. The mail was subjected to rigorous quarantine regulations. Officials in Sardis went beyond simple quarantine mail restrictions and prohibited any paper mail from entering the city's environs. Officials in Summit thoroughly fumigated all its mail before delivery. Many newspapers ceased publication or were reduced to listing the latest local deaths. Often, pertinent news did not reach towns because many local telegraph operators fell victim to the dreaded contagion. Many communities were isolated and fearful.

The deep-rooted fear of yellow fever frequently created bizarre events. In Columbus, Mississippi, law enforcement officials jailed a horse thief during the epidemic. While serving his time in September, he died of yellow fever. His unburied body remained in the jailhouse for three days, as no one would enter the jail cell for fear of contracting the disease.[45] In the coastal village of Handsboro, an elderly fisherman died in his small hut after contracting the disease. His decomposing body was found after a few days when townsfolk noticed that they had not seen him for a while. Again, because of fear of yellow fever, none of the locals would enter the hut to collect his body for burial, even with the offer of a generous reward. Instead, the townsfolk burned the hut with the fisherman's body inside. As one account stated, "the body of the old fisherman [was] reduced to ashes with the house."[46] In these two instances, people were still available to tell these tales. Most citizens, however, were so fearful of the disease that they fled when news broke in their region of any yellow fever cases. Further north in Grenada, J. P. Dromgoole reported that "every empty cabin, out-house, and church within eight or ten miles west of Grenada (and we suppose, in every other direction) has been occupied by families from town, living as best they may, and cut off from all communication with the settlers around. The country people are alarmed."[47] In short, most Mississippians were in a state of distress. Any semblance of normalcy had ceased to exist once yellow fever had begun its assault on the state.

6

Mississippi and the Affirmation of Antebellum Values

The circle steadily narrows.
—Jefferson Davis, *New York Herald,* October 22, 1878

The "normality" that appeared in Mississippi in 1878 was the reaffirmation of antebellum white social values—self-government, civic-mindedness, and a sense of duty on the part of white elites, with a concomitant racism toward African Americans. However, these values were weakened and proved to be ineffectual. By focusing on individual acts of heroism, white Mississippians could take pride in themselves even as "southern values" proved so ineffective in the epidemic. This was particularly clearly displayed in October 1878, as the disease spread to its widest geographical extent.

During that month, the more urban locales that had been first infected with the contagion began to experience a decline in both case and death numbers. However, health officials in the rural villages and crossroads began to record greater numbers of victims. Refugees fleeing the contagion in cities had more than likely carried yellow fever to the more rural parts of the state. Consequently, the pattern was one of constant infection and reinfection, thereby disrupting routine day-to-day activities during the month of October.[1]

The disease's appearance in locales once free from yellow fever created an even more panicked atmosphere because citizens in those areas had believed they were safe from the contagion, as had those who had fled to these regions. As ever, quarantines compounded the problem—they were either too lax to prevent spread of the disease or so strict that they paralyzed communities. Quarantines remained in effect through October, restricting both urban and rural activities, even as the mosquitoes slipped through lines of defense. Thus commercial interruptions continued in Mississippi, and many regions began to look to federal aid and continued distributions from Howard associations and other benevolent organizations to carry them through these difficult times. Federal aid played an increasingly important role as the epidemic continued into the fall months. Yet at no time does one find such an emphasis on civic duty resulting in homegrown heroism and mixed with affirmation of white antebellum values.

An important example of this phenomenon was Meridian, located in Lauderdale County in the eastern part of Mississippi. The town's population prior to the yellow fever epidemic was approximately three thousand. Local officials had taken prompt action, enacting early in the epidemic a pedestrian quarantine so severe that one contemporary stated that even a rat "could not get through without being detected." Perhaps as a result of the tight quarantine, Meridian had been "remarkably healthy" before the first week of October.[2]

In Meridian, as elsewhere in Mississippi, racism was deeply embedded in reporting about the disease, perhaps all the stronger for the experience of Reconstruction. Thus officials ignored the first yellow fever death, on September 24, that of the African American Lewis Carter. It was only when a white man, John Etheridge, died on September 28 that health officials acknowledged the fact that the city was experiencing yellow fever infection. Carter's case did not propel Meridian's health officials into action, but Etheridge's did. Etheridge had been a quarantine officer and a member of Lauderdale Masonic Lodge 308, so his position in Meridian's white society was well established. He left behind a wife and several children. The death of this prominent citizen crystallized the city's yellow fever fear. In an all-too-familiar pattern, "The people of the town now became panic stricken and a general stampede took place," reported J. L. Power. Most stores in Meridian closed as their proprietors fled to the countryside for safety. "Almost every one that could leave town did so," added another contemporary. Within days, only eight hundred citizens remained in Meridian, more than half of them African Americans.[3]

Although the state government gave no help, that did not mean that Meridian was helpless. White Mississippians had always placed a high value on civicmindedness, and prominent citizens had always been looked to for leadership. Nor, despite the heavy toll of war and Reconstruction, did people look in vain. Meridian's remaining white citizens organized an aid society, and four doctors volunteered to stay in town and treat the sick. Dr. George H. Fowler of Mobile also journeyed to Meridian during this time to help the stricken. Believing it to be their duty to stay behind to tend yellow fever victims, the mayor and three aldermen volunteered their services, as did the marshal, the sheriff, and the jailer. Two of them, both Masons, died in October as they ministered to the ailing. Alderman A. A. Currie, who had commanded a company in the Thirteenth Mississippi Regiment during the Civil War, "strictly attended to [his duty] until he was stricken down" by "the grim monster [that] laid his icy touch upon" him during the epidemic. Keenly aware of these men's Confederate and pre-Confederate allegiances, officials lamented their deaths and described their loss with rhetoric emphasizing the idealism of self-government and duty. These men exemplified the ideal that men in positions of prominence and authority were honor-bound to aid the helpless. Alderman William T. McLean owned a "flouring and meal mill" in Meridian and had offered his business's service free of charge to the afflicted city—at least the white helpless. He had also "stood to his post as a faithful sentinel during the epidemic, visiting the sick, feeding the hungry, and [was] always ready and willing to aid and assist those not able to help themselves."[4]

Nonetheless, after yellow fever was acknowledged publicly, any efforts of the civic-minded to help the white or African-American citizens were greatly hampered in Meridian because of the mass exodus of people and the pedestrian quarantine. On October 11, because of the rampant infection, even the trains stopped running through the town. For every prominent citizen who remained to do his or her duty, two or three members of the same elite appear to have fled. The president of the Meridian Aid Society manned the telegraph and transmitted "the gloomy story of suffering" as he also requested aid. Those who remained did their best to relieve the hardships of others—at least the whites—under the adverse conditions. Robert J. Moseley, a Mason and once sheriff of Lauderdale County, offered his house as a hospital for yellow fever cases. Moseley was "generous, true to his friends and liberal to a fault," epitomizing the ideal of self-help. However, he contracted the fever and died on October 9. As a result of further public appeals for aid, supplies finally began to pour into Meridian from the Masons as October continued. By October 18, however, there were 168 yellow fever cases and 48 recorded deaths. The *Pascagoula Democrat-Star* succinctly reported the situation in Meridian during this month by writing, "Disease spreading."[5]

But what of the black populace? The fact that few African Americans could afford to flee the disease left a strange situation in affected towns: the white elite that stayed from a sense of duty found itself check by jowl with former slaves. By the end of October, many Meridian households had suffered the loss of loved ones to Yellow Jack. The disease claimed seventy-five victims in the city during the month of October. Of those deaths, thirty-two were African Americans. This was a higher percentage of African-American yellow fever deaths than was usually recorded. Undoubtedly, since the majority of the white population had fled, the more likely victims were the African Americans who remained in the city. Research has not yielded the distribution of Masonic money between the remaining white and African-Americans citizens of the city. In October, monetary contributions amounted to $6,812 to help citizens of Meridian.[6]

A similar pattern appeared in Yazoo City in western Mississippi, where those who could do so had already fled by October; therefore, African Americans outnumbered whites by two to one. As with other Mississippi towns, Yazoo City recorded a drastic population decrease as yellow fever spread into its limits. The city's pre-epidemic population was approximately 2,500, but when the disease made its appearance that number dropped to 600. Of those, 200 were white and 400 were African American. The city had established quarantine restrictions on August 8 after hearing news of yellow fever's presence in other Mississippi locales. Officials quickly implemented the recommendations of the state board of health by disinfecting public places with a carbolic acid mixture and by fumigating the city and its environs with burning tar.[7]

When an African American violated quarantine, he or she was careless, criminal, or unclean; when a white person did the same, the act was often attributed to altruism. A case in point is the situation of St. Mary's Convent in Yazoo City. All six nuns housed at the convent contracted the disease. Father Mouton, the local Catholic priest, had to attend to their medical needs as well as those of others battling the disease. City officials attempted to quarantine the convent, but Father Mouton insisted upon being allowed to travel in and out of the religious house in order to care for the nuns. No public outcry arose against this flagrant disregard for recommended quarantine. A general unwillingness to restrict the movements of prominent citizens existed. However, this situation also presented a delicate situation, as the priest could not live at the convent to tend to the nuns: that would have been improper. On October 3, Father Mouton, who had cared diligently for those with yellow fever, died of the disease. Three of the six Sisters of Charity—Zenobia, Corona, and Mary Lawrence—also expired that day. Out of the seventeen total cases recorded in Yazoo City, nine deaths occurred; five of them were the dedicated priest, nuns of St. Mary's, and a Protestant minister. Most clergy believed it their Christian duty to offer health care and other services in stricken cities. At least one African American died of yellow fever in Yazoo City's epidemic. The deaths of some African Americans went unrecorded.[8]

Although newspapers usually tried to instill courage in readers, Dr. P. J. McCormick of the state board of health vehemently criticized the press for creating panic among citizens: "There was also an amount of alarm which I never witnessed before, due in a great measure to the reprehensible practice of filling the newspapers of the day with descriptions of the disease. To this, I think, may be attributed many deaths." The doctor did not specify how alarm over yellow fever resulted in deaths or if these incidents occurred exclusively in Yazoo City. His remarks are mystifying, as Yazoo City experienced fewer yellow fever deaths than other Mississippi locales. McCormick's observation probably pertained to events throughout the state as the contagion spread to regions previously unaffected—carried by refugees—and not just in Yazoo City.[9] Perhaps, though, the critic did not notice the large number of inspirational stories reported in loving detail.

Such inspirational tales were rarely told of African Americans, though. The arrival of fever in Jackson, the state capital, shows how eager white people were to point the finger of blame at African Americans. As with other locales stricken by yellow fever in October, officials in Jackson attempted to trace the origin of contagion. The *Jackson Clarion* reported on October 2 that yellow fever entered the city in September because Buck Patton, an African American, allowed his stepson from a "highly infected area" to come and live in Patton's Jackson home. Patton lived on the town square with his mother and family. His young stepson could have transported infected mosquitoes with him unknowingly, or he might have had a mild case of yellow fever that passed unrecognized. Within two weeks of his arrival, a young daughter of Patton's died of a disease that the attending physician said at the time had strongly marked yellow fever symptoms. However, another explanation for the source is that yellow fever had merely been milder in earlier instances; it could have been present in mosquitoes and subclinical individuals since the three cases in September. The editors of the local paper, who lambasted Patton's actions, would not have understood the disease's etiology. They were searching for a source to blame, and Patton, because he was an African American, was the easiest target to single out. Lashing out at Patton's apparent disregard for quarantine measures, the editors stated: "Fortunately for the rest of the community the sanitary measures enforced by the authorities delayed the progress of the disease, else our town would . . . have been enshrouded in the same gloom that has darkened so many other places. . . . We have no patience to comment upon the criminal violation of the ordinances which were established to protect the public health, and which, in addition to the punishment it has brought upon the parties who were accessory to it, has brought unspeakable sorrow upon at least one unfortunate family." Regardless of the source of contagion, Jackson would soon be "enshrouded" in yellow fever's gloom.[10]

Jackson newspapers also encouraged hope by watching carefully for signs of abatement. Once yellow fever invaded the city in October, it did so with a vengeance. One newspaper observed that "the death march" steadily continued into this "new field." By October 9 there were fifty-seven cases of yellow fever, with ten deaths recorded. "Fever on the increase" was the phrase continuously used to describe the situation in Jackson. On the nights of October 17, 18, and 19, however, a glimmer of hope appeared for the city when light frosts occurred. The local newspaper also reported a frost on October 22, while predicting that "unless nature has reversed her ordinances, cool weather will extinguish the disease ere long." Health officials, however, witnessed no decrease in the number of yellow fever cases and deaths, as one evening of light frost was not enough to kill the mosquitoes. On October 22, the same day that the temperature dipped below 32 degrees, officials recorded 350 cases of yellow fever in Jackson. The *Clarion* also noted in the previous day's edition that a large number of "colored" yellow fever cases existed in the city. This observation supports two interpretations. On the one hand, it is likely that fewer African Americans left Jackson when news of yellow fever reached the city, as they were too poor to flee and had nowhere to go. On the other hand, the phrase "a large number" reflects the careless record keeping concerning the African Americans' experience in the epidemic. Newspapers listed specific numbers for whites but were vague in reporting for African Americans, reaffirming that the press was for and by whites.[11]

Throughout October, Jackson's citizens, black and white, bore the weight of the yellow fever epidemic. Officials recorded 61 yellow fever deaths out of 416 reported cases. One citizen congratulated Jackson's "superb corps of able physicians" for maintaining expert standards of care and stated that "from the start [they] have contested every inch of ground with the fell destroyer." Of the 61 deaths, 33 were white and 28 were African American. Probably the most accurate observation regarding the epidemic in Jackson appeared in the *Clarion* on October 16. Editors stated that "Time at this season of the year is an important ally," referring to the advancing cold weather that eventually would kill the mosquitoes and their larvae. Frost usually occurred during October, and cold temperatures eventually slowed the fever's progress. Jackson and the rest of Mississippi could only await those dipping temperatures.[12]

Just as in other communities across Mississippi, Jacksonians reestablished or reaffirmed old social patterns as they fought the pestilence before cold weather set in. The *Clarion* reported the events of the epidemic in terms of battle, describing the doctors as fighting for "every inch of ground." Editors harkened back to the experiences of the Civil War, when Union forces left Jackson in ruins, regardless of the Confederates' valiant attempts to protect it.[13] Newspapers perpetuated that southern ethos throughout the epidemic.

White Mississippians were also prepared to recognize southern values in recent transplants to the South. Thus, in Scranton the death of Captain Patrick Mullett on October 11 evoked effusive praise. Mullett was from Lockport, New York, and had been working in Jackson County's shipping industry. The local paper's eloquent obituary stated that Mullett was "an upright, liberal and honest gentleman. Although but a short time in the South, . . . Capt. Mullett [had] won many warm friends . . . Poor Pat." Even though Mullett was not a native southerner, locals accepted him as one of their own.[14]

By the end of October, most communities in Jackson County appeared to be near the end of their bouts with yellow fever. Local papers jubilantly announced the closing stages of the epidemic and listed falling case and mortality figures. For example, Pascagoula had experienced seventeen cases since September 29, four proving fatal. Scranton officials reported even fewer, only five cases and three deaths. On October 11 the epidemic claimed its last victim in that town when Richard G. Davis, an architect and native of southern Wales, died of the disease.[15] These two cities in Jackson County experienced no further distress, but to the west, Ocean Springs still labored under the effects of yellow fever.

The situation in Ocean Springs, which recorded twenty-eight white deaths and one black casualty by the end of October, provided another opportunity to reaffirm values in the face of catastrophe. The fever appeared to affect mostly those at the local boardinghouses, where people roomed in close proximity to one another. Among the dead in that city were Colonel F. S. Strout, the proprietor of the Ocean Springs Hotel, and Father Charles from the local Catholic church, who died while ministering to the sick. Local reports surmised that when yellow fever first appeared in Ocean Springs, the "unacclimated" fell first, "but as material [victims] became exhausted, the spread began among local citizens." Of course, all citizens were at risk. Summarizing Ocean Springs's situation, the *Pascagoula Democrat-Star* reported on October 25: "To the east stood the forts of a rigid quarantine, to the west stretched a space of affliction, to the north a vast region of pines, to the south the ruffled waters of the gulf, but, thanks to the Throne above, *some* [local charities] knew our wants and sent relief to the destitute." This statement suggests that the security blanket of local responsibility was pretty thin and frayed—but the newspapers were doing all they could to patch it and recall people to their duty. Even so, by the end of October, Ocean Springs witnessed an end to the progress of the epidemic, and citizens of Jackson County breathed a collective sigh of relief.[16]

Regardless of Jackson County's atypically low case and death numbers in October, other coastal counties were still experiencing yellow fever's effects. Health officers at Mulatto Bayou in Hancock County verified one yellow fever case and death, and Pearlington officials recorded 201 cases and 24 deaths, with the majority in the Logtown region. In Bay St. Louis, two physicians were treating approximately forty to fifty cases of yellow fever, and by the end of October they verified seventy-eight fever deaths. Even though most towns in Hancock County had reported a considerable number of yellow fever victims, the epidemic appeared to have ended by the end of October. One reporter in Hancock County observed that "the panic is over. No more families are leaving."[17]

Harrison County, situated between Jackson and Hancock counties, also continued to report yellow fever's effects through October. Officials in Mississippi City commented that the town looked gloomy because of all of the sickness. Dr. John E. Lyon, a young physician from South Carolina who had married a woman from Handsboro, died on October 18.[18] Citizens in that small town noted that they had lost a devoted physician who had worked throughout the epidemic until he became sick with the fever. His death was certainly "melancholy news" to the people of Handsboro and Harrison County. Regardless, the proprietors of the Tegarden and Barnes hotels both indicated that the numerous yellow fever sufferers staying there were recovering. However, the Barnes Hotel announced that it would close its doors on October 5, since officials had confirmed twenty-one cases in and near the public house. In one newspaper's obituary column on October 4, six yellow fever deaths from Handsboro appeared out of nine cases reported. Three of the victims were from the Murphy family. John and Emma Murphy, a young couple living in the Handsboro region, had two daughters, Mary Jane, age three, and Catherine, six months. The couple watched helplessly as the girls died of yellow fever, Mary Jane on October 7 and Catherine on October 9. John Murphy then stood by powerlessly when on October 16 Emma died.[19]

The case of Jefferson Davis, former president of the Confederacy, and his family illustrates the preferential treatment and focus of attention on the prominent in this post-Reconstruction world and affirms an image of the "true" white Mississippian. When news of the crisis reached Jefferson and Varina Davis at their home Beauvoir, located east of Handsboro on the Gulf of Mexico, both were unwell and unable to flee. Davis had fallen ill during his post–Civil War imprisonment, and both of them were aged and too weak to travel. Both had wanted to escape to Memphis to be with their daughter Margaret and her husband, J. Addison Hayes. Their son Jefferson Davis Jr. was also in Memphis, living with his sister and working with his brother-in-law at the State National Bank of Memphis. When the yellow fever epidemic broke out, Margaret moved six miles outside Memphis into the countryside for her safety. Hayes and Jefferson Jr. traveled back into Memphis every day in order to maintain the bank's operations. Hayes had petitioned Washington, D.C., for permission to move the bank's assets to Nashville, but permission had been denied. Therefore, Hayes, an accountant, and Jefferson Jr. maintained business activities at the bank, believing it to be their duty to their fellow citizens.[20]

Writing to Margaret on September 25, Jefferson Davis Sr. expressed how proud he was of his son's sense of duty as he helped people with their banking needs: "of course, I honor the devotion to duty which has led him to stand to his post as long as it was needful to hold it."[21] He apparently had no doubts that his son would fulfill his duty to the citizens of Memphis during this dire time. Jefferson Jr. was dedicated to his sister and also quite fond of his brother-in-law. Even though the men fumigated themselves every evening before returning home to Margaret, Jefferson Jr. contracted yellow fever. He refused to allow his sister to enter his room for fear that she, too, might catch the disease. During his sickness, Dr. Robert Mitchell, the head of the Memphis Howards, traveled out and tended to him every day, accompanied by two Sisters of Charity, demonstrating a clear favoritism for the prominent. Nothing, however, could save him, and on October 10, Jefferson Davis Jr. died of yellow fever.[22]

Thus, the Davises lost their only remaining son to the disease. The Memphis and Charleston Railroad arranged for a train car and engine to be at their disposal, but the couple was too feeble to travel. Local newspapers announced along the coast, "by dispatches from Memphis . . . that Jefferson Davis, Jr., son of ex-President Davis, died . . . of yellow fever." Margaret arranged for his burial in Elmwood Cemetery in Memphis. Even though Davis senior did not attend his son's funeral, he was well represented by friends and admirers. The "reverential sympathy felt by all the true hearted of his countrymen" honored the senior Davis. The Presbyterian clergyman in attendance, Rev. Dr. Boggs, offered a prayer "for the afflicted family . . . in a voice broken with emotion and accompanied by uncontrollable evidences of the feelings of the bystanders." According to accounts, the emotionalism of this funeral was overwhelming, even during this terrible scourge when death was so commonplace. During this epidemic, southerners had a tendency to channel feelings through the prominent so that even Jefferson Davis's son became an icon of southern heroism.[23]

The death of Jefferson Davis's last remaining son had an impact on many others besides the immediate family. The Davis family embodied the ideals of southern honor and duty, according to contemporaries, and the son of the former Confederate president would have epitomized a southern gentleman. By the time of the epidemic, the South had already begun to commemorate the southern soldiers who had died in the Civil War. According to one account, Mrs. Charles J. Williams of Columbus, Georgia, first decorated the graves of Confederate casualties in her area in 1868, thereby beginning Confederate Memorial Day and eventually, National Memorial Day. Regardless of its origins, the idea of Decoration Day or Confederate Memorial Day, still celebrated in nine southern states, including Mississippi, perpetuated the memory and ideals of what ultimately became known as the "Lost Cause." By 1878 the Davis family, and especially Jefferson Jr., symbolized that recognition of lost culture; therefore, the younger Davis's death affected not only his family but also those who looked to this family for symbolic representation of southern honor and duty, even through the epidemic.[24]

Many less-prominent Mississippi men received the same sort of idolization. In Holly Springs, reporter W. J. L. Holland volunteered to help during the epidemic. Chairman of the city's relief committee, he continued to offer his services even as that organization underwent two complete personnel changes because of its members' deaths, as most of the first round of members died in the epidemic. For a time, Holland was the only member of the committee who was able to minister to the citizens of Holly Springs. He was thirty-six years old when he died of yellow fever on October 25. The *Holly Springs Reporter* lamented "the death of our associate and dear friend, . . . who fell at his post, ministering to the wants of the sick and dying in the recent epidemic." His death created "a void in our heart, and in the heart of this community, that cannot be filled," concluded the eulogy.[25]

The fact that Holland contracted yellow fever after the first frost in Holly Springs made his death even more disturbing, as many believed that he had outlasted the scourge that had raged during the epidemic's first two months. Mississippians knew that frost signaled the end of the plague and the return of safety. Holland's death at the end of October troubled many in Holly Springs, especially members of the Bonner family who had recently buried their own dead. Kate McDowell wrote to her friend and mentor Henry Wadsworth Longfellow that news of Holland's death "seems almost unendurable. He was the last of those noble young men who voluntarily gave their lives." She had hoped that he would survive the warning signs of yellow fever, but on October 25 that "sudden dreadful symptom that always heralds death [black vomit]" appeared. McDowell and her family were especially saddened by Holland's death, since her sister, Lilly, had been engaged to him.

Similar "brightest spirits" continued to fall to yellow fever in Vicksburg through October, by which time the city was virtually a town of death as only doctors, nurses, and health officials traveled there to help the sick and dying. St. Paul's Catholic Church remained open as a refuge for those with the disease. Father John McManus and his assistant, Father John Vitolo, both died of yellow fever along with four Sisters of Mercy. One, Sister Mary Regis, was from Copiah County, Mississippi, and had just entered the convent on February 23, 1878. Sister Mary Bernadine Murray was also a recent arrival to the convent, having entered on December 21, 1877. Both worked tirelessly ministering to the suffering citizens of Vicksburg until they, too, lay among the victims. Another member of the order, Sister Mary Vincent, traveled to Meridian with a small group "to bring peace and comfort to the parting soul" of all who died of yellow fever. Because of the shotgun quarantine in place, she was unable to complete the trip between Vicksburg and Meridian. The conductor of the train forced the nuns to disembark ten miles from Meridian at the small village of Chunky, since the train could not enter the city. The women received warm hospitality at Chunky until they finally made their way back to Vicksburg. Sister Mary Vincent survived the 1878 epidemic.[26]

In Vicksburg, diarists recorded their fears as they weathered the epidemic. Sophie Adams Goodrum described the deaths of two of her closest friends, Patience Kline and Theresa Nailer, who died within two days of one another in early October. Fearing that they would contract the disease from those who had died of yellow fever, townspeople buried both women in the evening hours on the same day they died. Goodrum wrote that Klein was like a sister to her, but because of her disease, she and others were "afraid to enter her sick room, and listen to her last words of wisdom." As in the case of Lilly McDowell in Holly Springs, many physicians and citizens believed that others could contract yellow fever through contact with the sick. Citizens in Vicksburg and other towns sometimes died alone because family and friends feared contracting the disease.[27]

Dread of the contagion occasionally caused normal people to react abnormally. One contemporary source described the panic among citizens around Vicksburg as "worse than that among a routed army." Dr. R. H. Ferry recounted that absolute fear motivated the parents of two dying children to abandon them to the care of strangers, an act that demonstrated a lack of adherence to the southern values exhibited by many during the epidemic. After the children died, African Americans buried them out of the kindness of their hearts, according to Ferry.[28]

During October approximately 136 people died of yellow fever in Vicksburg, including the nuns and priests. Of that number, 105 were white and 31 were African American. Earnest Hardenstein, however, noted that "the poorer class . . . particularly the blacks, buried their own dead." The city sexton, therefore, did not possess all of the records, so these numbers are only approximations. This accounting problem with people in authority was common regarding African Americans throughout Mississippi.[29]

During the epidemic, when Mississippians first turned to the state for aid, little was forthcoming. That they even sought aid suggests that a new idea of the sphere of government involvement had taken root. But it did not last long in the face of government impotence. The state government was hamstrung because it had not appropriated adequately funds to its state board of health and had not set aside any relief funds. Therefore, agencies like the Howards provided help after communities requested it; nuns and other religious professionals, already in the communities, also quickly organized relief efforts. Like the Masons, the Howards had both local and interstate branches. As a result, these two groups provided impressive aid to the state. Regardless of the number of relief associations and individuals ministering to and caring for the sick, the numbers were too overwhelming.

In towns all over Mississippi the local elites requested help during the epidemic, acknowledging that the problem was too big for them to handle alone. In Harrison County, officials in Handsboro called for "money and nurses for the indigent poor and needy." C. Taylor, president of the local Howard Association, acted as the treasurer and disbursement agent for the funds for the Handsboro Howards.[30] These men reported to the state board of health and the local newspaper that they were doing all they could for the victims of yellow fever in their areas but that they still needed outside help, whether in the form of personnel, food, or money. To the east, Pascagoula did not need provisions but requested Howard workers. That city's officials convened a volunteers' meeting at B. J. Jane's restaurant to organize their local association better. Further north, Canton's relief committee needed "money, sugar, coffee, flour, rice and meat." Vicksburg's grand master of the Masons issued an additional appeal "to all Masons to contribute to the relief of the sick and destitute of this city."[31] As the epidemic progressed, towns could no longer rely upon their own resources. To cope with the tremendous economic pressure caused by the epidemic, locales interacted with one another in efforts to relieve their citizens. Therefore, communities that had once been isolated now became integrated into a larger regional and eventually national system of market interaction, including means of communication and transportation.

What outside assistance was acceptable and how people expressed their gratitude was also channeled into a reaffirmation of Mississippi values. The Howards maintained their high standard of medical relief, including sending large numbers of workers to provide nursing care, and the Masons and Odd Fellows in Mississippi continued to work closely with the Howards. In fact, J. L. Power, the grand secretary of Masons and grand treasurer of Odd Fellows, stated that if he was not directly able to give contributions to his benevolent orders, he sent the monies to the Howards, who had been "zealously co-operating" with the two other benevolent civic organizations. Power and the Masons maintained that aid should be given "regardless of race, color or class." For the purpose of distributing this assistance, the telegraph companies gave "free use of the wires, the express companies mark every package [for free shipment], the banks charge no discount or exchange, and the railroads carry supplies, nurses and doctors all free of charge."[32] During October, Mississippians were the recipients of munificent aid and philanthropic gestures. The Howards unflinchingly continued to answer the pleas of ordinary citizens during that month. As an organization with roots in the South, the Howards showed that there was substance behind the rhetoric of a glorious, noble South. Doctors and nurses journeyed to stricken locales across the state as politicians occupied themselves with power maneuvers.

In response to the Howards' relief outpourings, Mississippi's populace expressed gratitude in various ways, including tributes and specially chosen gifts. One example was the anonymous poem "The Howards of the South," which appeared in papers across the nation. It recounts the "brave hands that bear up nobly the stricken fevered head" and thanks the North for sending "her treasure, her silver and her gold, [but] you give your time, your courage and sympathy untold." The *London Standard* also printed a tribute that immortalized the

Howards as "the flower and pride of the great English race, on whom a more terrible, more merciless enemy has now fallen." The South's youth, according to the London tribute, "volunteer to serve and die in the plague-stricken cities," and "their sisters and wives, mothers and daughters, are dying and suffering" in towns "desolated by the yellow fever." The article further reported that nurses who volunteered to be Howards faced a "martyr's death." Tributes to the Howards also came in other forms. In Grenada, the local head of the Howard Association, D. W. Coon, received a gold watch from the citizens of that city for his selfless service during the epidemic. Commenting on the generosity of the members of the Howard Association and others, President Rutherford B. Hayes stated in his annual address to Congress: "The suffering and destruction that resulted excited the deepest sympathy in all parts of the Union. Physicians and nurses hastened from every quarter to the assistance of the afflicted communities. Voluntary contributions of money and supplies in every needed form were speedily and generously furnished."[33] The Howards were integral to the healing of Mississippi during the epidemic.

However, the Howards were not welcome in every Mississippi locality during the epidemic. Stonewall, a small community north of Biloxi on the Tchoutacabouffa River, reported only one yellow fever victim in its area by October 18. A representative of the Ocean Springs Howard Association journeyed to that village to ascertain if any medical or relief assistance was needed. Demonstrating zealous self-reliance, the people of Stonewall apparently felt insulted by the Howards' investigation, because on October 18 city officials observed in a local paper that "when we need assistance we will apply for it."[34] This was one of the few instances when aid from the Howards was rejected.

Certainly, the Howards reaffirmed southern values as self-reliant providers, an appreciated and accepted male sphere. Thus female Howard workers were paid much less than males, and African Americans received the least of all as representatives of marginal groups in society. Although the Howards provided aid to the majority of stricken areas in Mississippi, the nurses they hired usually experienced exasperating circumstances as they assisted the sick. Poor sanitary conditions and the nature of yellow fever symptoms made ministering to the stricken an overwhelming task, and compensation for nursing care probably was not commensurate with the job at hand. Nurses received far lower salaries than physicians did, even though both risked their lives equally to treat the sick. Physicians hired by the Howards earned ten dollars per day, with a horse and buggy provided, while nurses received four dollars per day with room and board. Black nurses hired by the Howards fared even worse, earning only three dollars per day with board. Perhaps because of the low pay and the frustration that accompanied nursing duty, one white nurse stationed at Hernando penned a letter to the Memphis Howard Association that had hired her to work in Mississippi. She stated that she was starving and that she was "broken down for want of food and rest." Her patient was a stern taskmaster: "Quinn will die, but he is so aggravating that he may live for two or three days; he has no friends, and no wonder, for a more cantankerous cuss I never met with." She was also unhappy about her location: "The folks at the rum-mill above are only swine and will not come near me." In a plea for help, she ended her letter by threatening: "I am sick and starving, and in self-defense will have to leave or kill the patient, and I do not like to do either. Come at once or I leave." Although this woman was not typical of the nurses who worked for the Howards, she was not shy about complaining that compensation was not adequate for her demanding nursing job and that her room and board were substandard. The outcome of the situation between Quinn and his nurse remains unknown, but no Quinn appears in Power's or Keating's lists of yellow fever deaths for Hernando.[35]

At every level, Mississippians attempted to ease the stresses of those affected by the yellow fever epidemic. Catholics helped Catholics; Protestants helped Protestants; Jews helped Jews. Prominent white organizations like the Odd Fellows' Relief Committee, the Masonic Relief Organization, the Knights of Pythias Relief Committee, the Knights of Honor, and the Printers' Relief Committee helped those less fortunate. In Vicksburg, concerned citizens organized the Catholic Orphan Relief Association to identify and care for Catholic children left without parents in that city and the surrounding countryside. Each ward of the town had its own committee head whose job was to maintain statistics regarding children whose parents died of yellow fever. On October 7 the city's Protestants established a counterpart to the Catholic association, the Committee for Orphans, which focused on Protestant children of any denomination whose parents died in the epidemic. The unusual aspect of the Committee for Orphans was that its members were all female, illustrating further women's roles as caregivers in this epidemic. Additionally, a Jewish committee mobilized in Vicksburg to provide relief for anyone of that faith needing assistance. The Printers' Relief Committee was exclusively for members of Vicksburg's Typographical Union. Of all these groups, however, the Howards and the Masons were the only ones who did not discriminate according to race, sex, creed, or social position.

When it became apparent that Mississippi could not provide adequately for its own citizens, appeals for outside help became numerous. Help came, but it was never enough. In Mississippi towns it was the federal government that eventually stepped in to help, not the state. The U.S. Army donated rations to aid the stricken regions of Mississippi. The federal government also organized relief efforts at this time to get provisions to the state's stricken areas. As the South continued to deal with the epidemic, it became apparent that southerners could not go it alone. Monies and medical workers were already providing assistance, but the epidemic was too overwhelming. Therefore, the U.S. Congress assembled a crew and outfitted the *John M. Chambers* to ply the Mississippi River and distribute goods.

When the federal government got involved in disaster relief, its efforts were only partly acceptable, thanks to the dynamics of Mississippi white "honor." Mississippians, like other southerners, remembered federal intrusion during Reconstruction; therefore they were often wary of federal aid, fearing the consequences of accepting government relief. Republican president Rutherford B. Hayes, elected in 1876, nevertheless recognized the dire yellow fever situation in the South and saw that the disease had caused "an emergency which called for prompt and extraordinary measures of relief. . . . The states of Louisiana, Mississippi, and Tennessee have suffered severely."[36] Consequently, the U.S. Congress created a Yellow Fever National Relief Commission on September 11, 1878, to receive and distribute donations collected for stricken citizens in yellow fever areas. Alexander R. Shepherd was the chairman of that executive committee, which had eleven other members, including a secretary and a treasurer.[37]

After collecting and organizing a relief party, the National Relief Commission appointed Lieutenant Hiram H. Benner to pilot the relief boat, the *John M. Chambers,* down the Mississippi River. Benner was to distribute provisions to Mississippians during October from this three-hundred-ton stern-wheeler, stopping at various ports in the state. On October 4 the *Chambers* and its crew began their relief journey with a surgeon, a druggist, servicemen from the Thirteenth and Eighteenth U.S. Infantry, and correspondents for Chicago and St. Louis newspapers. The ship also carried twenty carbines and two thousand rounds of ammunition in case mobs attacked the boat as it made its stops. Although no such riots in Mississippi are recorded, the federal government had little trust in Mississippians' rationality and self-control. Because the *Chambers* carried food and clothing supplies that parts of the South (including Mississippi) had not had access to for approximately three months, northern officials were worried about an attack on the vessel. Stores on board the ship included needles, coffins, rice, molasses, grits, candles, tea, sugar, snuff, flour, clam chowder, and canned tomatoes. The range of goods also included shoes, "drawers," socks, pillow ticks, and dressing gowns. Also, the supply of ice on board the ship facilitated food preservation and cold storage for corpses awaiting burial.[38]

As the *Chambers* chugged down the Mississippi, it stopped at the river towns to distribute its bounty. Arriving at Friar's Point on October 8, officers from the boat entrusted Mayor T. S. Aderbolt with 1,023 pounds of ice and a box of lemons. Later that day the crew unloaded 250 pounds of ice at Terrene, in Bolivar County. That city had only twelve cases of yellow fever and four deaths, so officials must have decided its needs were not as great as other locations'. The next day, the *Chambers* pulled in to Greenville, where Rev. Stevenson Archer was waiting at the wharf to meet the relief vessel and conduct the transfer of goods. Many items were left for the suffering citizens of Greenville, including six coops of chickens, flour, onions, coffee, clothes, lard, and ten tons of ice. After leaving that locale, the boat continued to Port Gibson and Grand Gulf, arriving on October 12. Jasper A. Gage, the president of the Howard Association in Port Gibson, received massive quantities of household items, food, and clothing earmarked for relief aid and estimated at a value of $5,000. He was to distribute the goods equitably among the populace. The directive to Gage suggests a federal concern about the inclusion of non-elites and African Americans in relief efforts. Included in the donations were two dozen lead pencils that were not listed in the original boat manifest. The captain of the *Chambers* reserved the remainder of the boat's cargo for the citizens of Vicksburg, docking there on October 13. W. H. Andrews, president of the local Howard Association, supervised the unloading, counting, and distribution of the goods. Lieutenant Benner transferred all provisions to the Howards with apparent confidence that the organization would complete the distribution of the humanitarian aid.[39]

At least some whites did not want to give anything to African Africans, and resented federal orders that they should do so. The problem was clear in Vicksburg, where controversy arose between the white and black populations about how to divide relief provisions. Harsh criticism of African Americans appeared when the *Vicksburg Weekly Herald* argued that large numbers of African Americans "who toil not" but "subsist in luxurious ease and idleness on the liberality of the Northern people, and the beneficence of the Howard Association" should not receive any more goods. "All over the Southland the fields are whitening with cotton ready for the picker, and yet these able-bodied healthy men and women stand here in Vicksburg and draw free rations," the article concluded.[40] The true reason for this attack was that white landowners lacked workers to pick their cotton. The editors, however, clarified that they did not want to appear opposed to relief being extended to the "colored people, but we are not in favor of them, or anyone else, being allowed to subsist in idleness upon the supplies so generously donated to the sick and destitute of our stricken county."[41] White Mississippians in positions of authority appeared more than willing to accept federal assistance as long as they were able to control how and to whom the aid was given. Perhaps because they themselves were unable to provide the needed assistance, they sought to preserve some degree of perceived autonomy.

E. Cordwent, a refugee from the South who was waiting in Chicago for the fever to abate, added his response to the previous week's editorial in the *Vicksburg Weekly Herald:* "I see as usual when they think [they] can get anything without working for it, the negroes are flocking to town to get free rations." This suggests evidence of deep-seated racial resentment. Now, with a Democratic state government in place and little federal pressure, that bitterness could be expressed more freely. Apparently, Cordwent had been in contact with someone at his farm in the Vicksburg area, for he assured the public that "every negro on my place is supplied with all the rations necessary, and I hope if any of them applies for rations that you will not furnish it." Cordwent is stressing that he has the ability to care for his "people" under his control, just as any patriarch in antebellum Mississippi would have done. His resentment toward outside aid is obvious. Also, it is logical to assume that Cordwent's workers charged their necessities at his commissary as was still the custom of the day on large landholdings in the South, so of course he would be upset if goods were distributed without charge. However, and more importantly, by accepting outside aid for the African Americans under his hegemony, Cordwent would have to recognize that he was not in control of his own affairs and thus was not able to perform as a strong patriarch. This was unacceptable to many white Mississippians who had only recently been brought back into the Union after the Civil War. The editors also strongly suggested that "the better class of the colored people direct their influence and attention to the protection of the Howard Association from these oft recurring impositions by stout and hearty colored men."[42]

Disputes over aid distribution occurred in other locales as well. George E. Hasie reported from Newton that the rations sent to his region from Vicksburg went to no one "who either needed or deserved them." People "flocked with their baskets and sacks to the depot of distribution to demand their share. It is not needed, and only encourages them in laziness."[43] Hasie, Cordwent, and the editors at the *Vicksburg Weekly Herald* exemplified the racist policies of white landowners, who relied upon black labor but chose to ignore the abject poverty of most rural African Americans during this time.

The opinions expressed in 1878 mirrored attitudes expressed in 1874 about relief aid to African Americans. In 1874 a disastrous Mississippi River flood caused major damage to the Mississippi Delta. African Americans were especially hard pressed for aid during the late spring months as waters covered any hopes of successful crops. Just as during the 1878 epidemic, critics claimed that misappropriation of rations occurred, especially by African Americans.[44] There is no evidence to support these claims, however; it appears that these opinions were part of a general expression of outrage against the idea that the African Americans were entitled to anything, especially if it meant whites had to do without or were not involved in the decision-making process. Prejudices against relief aid to African Americans, therefore, were not unique; racial biases simply became magnified because of the epidemic's extent. According to historian Ted Ownby,

African Americans living in the southern countryside operated in an economic structure of "hard and steady labor." Their living conditions were spartan at best, and white supremacist landowners often echoed E. Cordwent's opinions. Undoubtedly, no African American lived in "luxurious ease" as a result of outside assistance during this epidemic, or for that matter before it. Until African Americans in Mississippi could participate in wage work in industries other than agriculture, economic conditions for them would be difficult. During trying times, those already constructed tensions became even more prominent as goods became scarce and structures of social control were strained.[45]

In reaction to racial tension during the yellow fever epidemic, African Americans in Vicksburg organized their own relief organization, the Peabody Association, possibly patterning and naming their agency after the Peabody Subsistence Association in New Orleans.[46] The latter group distributed aid to New Orleanians who needed provisions during the yellow fever epidemic; however, it was a white group. The Vicksburg organization elected George W. Stith as president and Thomas M. Broadwaters as treasurer. On October 10, Stith complained that the African Americans in Vicksburg had contributed to the Howards but that they were not getting their fair share of aid. Similar complaints also appeared in New Orleans and Memphis during the 1878 epidemic. In Vicksburg, the Howard Association was upset over this accusation and requested an investigation into the allegations by Lieutenant Benner of the docked *Chambers*. At the time of the request Lieutenant Benner was ill, so Lieutenant Charles S. Hall, the second in command, conducted the inquest.[47]

All parties involved in the controversy convened aboard the *Chambers*. Lieutenant Hall asked Stith if he knew "of a single case of sickness or destitution among the colored people, which had been reported to the Howards, which had not been promptly attended to." Stith could not provide an example of negligence, and Hall continued, "Don't you believe if you make your wants known to the Howards they will supply you with what you want?" Finally, after requesting that the Peabody group trust the "wisdom" of the Howard Association in the distribution of the *Chambers*'s supplies, Hall and Stith arrived at an agreement: the Peabody Association would help the Howards find cases of sickness or destitution among the black population in Vicksburg. The Peabody group received assurances that the Howards would "not discriminate on account of race or condition."[48] Apparently, officials intimidated Stith into a truce, or perhaps the fact that the epidemic was finally waning helped because the controversy over equitable relief distribution in Vicksburg did not appear again in the press for the duration of the epidemic. Race relations in post-Reconstruction Mississippi were strained, to say the least, and this event could have resulted in a major confrontation. Perhaps the mediation by federal forces and the fact that the do-nations of provisional aid came from the federal government resulted in an at-mosphere more conducive to compromise. It is even more likely that the Peabody Association felt free to complain and expect an investigation because this was the federal government and not the state of Mississippi.

Lieutenant Hall was successful in mediating between the two factions in Vicksburg, but Lieutenant Benner was not as lucky. Local newspapers reported that "the hot hand of the demon which stalks . . . in our midst, relentlessly as the rain which falls upon the just and unjust," had grabbed Lieutenant Benner. His case appeared extremely virulent from the outset. Despite receiving good nursing care, Benner died on October 17 in Vicksburg. Former Confederate and Union soldiers escorted his body to Genellas Hall in the city, where it lay in state until his funeral. From all accounts, visitors flocked to the building to pay their respects to Benner, both African Americans and whites waiting for hours to pass his coffin. His death created "a sensation more profound than could have been anticipated in a community whose capacity for suffering was supposed to have been long since exhausted." Three important clerics, including the Epis-copal bishop of Mississippi and two other ministers, officiated at Benner's fu-neral service. The Firemen's Silver Cornet Band played "The Funeral March of '78," composed for the occasion by Professor Peter Rivinac, who had been the bandmaster for the Twenty-eighth Mississippi Cavalry Regiment during the Civil War. The Vicksburg Howard Association paid for the funeral. City of-ficials buried Benner in the National Cemetery in Vicksburg. Citizens in this once-Confederate Mississippi River bastion demonstrated genuine affection and heartfelt sympathy for the federal officer who had provided some relief from the yellow fever suffering. Benner's funeral was an opportunity for southerners and northerners to "experience, articulate, and perform reconciliation."[49]

The remaining crew members of the *Chambers* further eulogized Benner when they organized an official resolution of condolence to Benner's wife and children. "The country has lost one of its noble defender[s], the army a brave, faithful and trusty officer, society a courteous gentleman, and his wife and chil-dren a devoted husband and father," they wrote. The officers and crew requested of reporters that the resolution be printed in the *St. Louis Globe-Democrat,* the *Atlanta Constitution,* and the *Vicksburg Weekly Herald.* Obviously, Benner's death from yellow fever affected Vicksburg and his command profoundly. Benner died helping the stricken South, serving those Mississippians who had suffered untold horrors. His story, therefore, touched all hearts, northern and southern.[50]

During October, relief efforts were plentiful as the epidemic began to wane. Suffering continued, but Mississippians in fever-stricken areas were able to think about returning to their normal life routines. Frost appeared in several locations by the end of the month, and most people assumed that the fever would finally abate as the cold weather crept into the state. Jack Frost would work his proven cure, and the citizens of Mississippi would be grateful and relieved even though they were unaware of why frost actually halted the spread of yellow fever. The epidemic was finally ending.

7
Yellow Fever Departs

There were not windows enough in the church to have memorials for all the
members who perished.

—*New York Herald,* November 11, 1878

When November arrived, yellow fever continued its withdrawal from Mississippi, and by December only sporadic cases and deaths occurred in the state.
Citizens, weary with the past three months of stress, finally heard sighs of relief
over the disease's departure. During the last two months of 1878, frost appeared
across the state somewhat regularly, particularly in the more northern regions
where some epidemic pockets still existed. Mississippians anxiously awaited the
prolonged periods of colder weather that usually heralded the end of the scourge.
As one commentator stated, "Thank God for the cold and frost. When Jack
Frost meets Yellow Jack then comes the tug of war. The two Jacks have met, and
Yellow Jack is dead."[1]

Even with the lower temperatures, relief disbursement in Mississippi continued
during these two months, particularly in November. By December, however,
only scattered monetary and commodity aid arrived. The majority of humanitarian funds had already been donated and received in the previous epidemic
months. Federal aid dispersed in October had not been adequate to meet the
needs of all affected people. For example, the *Chambers* carried only three hundred coffins on its Mississippi River run. This was not enough for one town, and
certainly not adequate for the entire region. Limited relief at this stage suggests
that Mississippians experienced an ongoing sense of isolation and alienation.
Many Mississippians probably needed more long-term relief efforts in order to
recover completely. However, citizens who were attempting to reestablish some
semblance of normalcy in their everyday lives still appreciated the material goods
and monetary relief as the epidemic waned.

As store owners and consumers returned to their homes, businesses began
to operate more regularly across the state. Officials in most communities lifted
quarantines for railroad, water, and pedestrian traffic during November; therefore, by December, commerce resumed quickly. Trains again carried necessary
goods and merchandise into the towns to stock depleted or recently closed stores.

As refugees returned to their homes throughout Mississippi, they needed goods that had been inaccessible during the months they sought safety elsewhere, particularly if they were not the recipients of or had no access to federal relief efforts in Mississippi River towns. Local newspapers welcomed their towns' return to normalcy as editors listed the names of survivors coming home and advertised stores' renewed commerce. Most citizens now breathed sighs of relief instead of despair as the business atmosphere quickly became brisk and routine daily schedules resumed.

For many, the paramount issue now became how to keep such a thing from ever happening again. Medical journals throughout the Southeast and beyond offered a professional site for physicians to voice their opinions regarding yellow fever's causes, treatments, and prevention. The southern medical community certainly desired to avoid another disastrous yellow fever epidemic; therefore, medical personnel debated the issues through their articles and commentary. Physicians from Mississippi probably read the opinions of their southern colleagues as they helped the state board of health prepare a truer picture of their own state's experience. For example, Dr. R. W. Mitchell of Memphis prescribed forcing the yellow fever patient to vomit and then administering ten to twelve grains of calomel. An empty stomach apparently facilitated quicker absorption rates for the drug. Mitchell also advocated mustard footbaths to accompany this prescription. The relation between the oral ingestion of calomel and a mustard footbath was not specified.[2]

Dr. L. P. Yandell of Louisville asserted that yellow fever spread to his region because of unsanitary conditions, particularly in Nicholson pavement. Nicholson pavement, made from cypress blocks set in pitch, absorbed any putrefying matter discarded in the open streets, thus creating a most odiferous and unhealthy condition. The pavement reeked with "putrid vegetable and animal matter." Yandell did not offer a preventative for yellow fever transmission, but his recommendation that Nicholson pavement be replaced could have affected the life cycle of *Aedes aegypti* mosquitoes, since they prefer small, stagnant pools of water for breeding, and ridding a town of pavement that collected water would have been helpful. Other reporting physicians, particularly in Memphis, listed Nicholson pavement as a possible source of contagion. Aware that calomel and quinine had been ineffectual in 1853 as well as during the 1878 epidemic, Dr. J. R. Uhler of Baltimore made an unusual recommendation for prevention: healthy persons should smear their bodies with "plenty of thick fat, such as lard or some common oil" to block the contagion from entering the body through the pores. In addition, all food should, according to Uhler, be liquefied so that it could be sucked through a straw, thereby avoiding any yellow fever contamination. Cotton wadding was also advised in order to cover food, resulting in a sterile field.

In retrospect, a "thick fat" body smear would have been an effective deterrent to mosquito bites.[3]

As the epidemic waned, physicians practicing in other parts of the country also published similar ideas in professional journals. Dr. H. D. Schmidt asserted in the *New York Medical Journal* that the correct means of yellow fever prevention was to find an "agent to effectively destroy yellow-fever poison adhering to clothes and other effects of people or to merchandise brought in ships without damage to these objects themselves." Schmidt realized that "without such an agent it is impossible to establish a quarantine both efficient and, at the same time, not interfering seriously with the interests of commerce." He also suggested four agents that could destroy yellow fever: ozone, ventilation, dry heat, and sunlight.[4] Despite numerous articles discussing the causes, treatments, and prevention of yellow fever, the medical community still did not understand the origin of the disease or its method of transmission. Medical practitioners commonly accepted the portability of yellow fever after the 1878 epidemic, because its course could be traced along railroad lines and water routes as refugees escaped along them. Dr. J. P. Davidson of New Orleans acknowledged the significance of railroad travel during the epidemic: "Heretofore the disease had followed the water-course in its dissemination[.] [T]his year it has traveled by rail, and the fear is that rapid intercommunication hereafter may be a fruitful source of its reaching distant communities."[5] The contemporary germ theory, with fomites as the method of transmission, also became acceptable to the majority of physicians as technological improvements such as more advanced use of the microscope provided further information for an alternative explanation of the nature of diseases. The idea that yellow fever had a living causative agent was generally replacing earlier etiological explanations. No longer were miasmic inhalations from swamps or putrid privies believed to be the cause of yellow fever. After the epidemic, most in the medical community appeared to believe that yellow fever was not contagious from person to person. They still grappled with divergent theories of treatment, however. It would not be until the 1880s that Dr. Carlos Finlay of Cuba experimented with mosquitoes as vectors in yellow fever transmission. By 1905, Finlay's mosquito theory would be proven.[6]

As the 1878 yellow fever epidemic wound down, the Mississippi State Board of Health continued to work closely with county and municipal boards of health, requesting information from those officials.[7] It also convened a year later, in November 1879, to analyze the medical information of stricken locales in the epidemic. The board needed official case numbers and deaths from those areas. Health and government officials within the state wanted to compile these statistics so that a better understanding of the disease's impact would be available. A more accurate accounting of the epidemic would expose the devastation of

1878 yellow fever experience. Physicians across the state submitted their findings to the state board of health. Throughout the epidemic months the board had offered numerous suggestions as to the best method for fumigation and had urged the establishment of quarantine restrictions, but it had been able to do little else. Collecting statistics was one function it could complete. Because it lacked legislative power, Mississippi's health board was unable to mandate any public health regulations, particularly in regard to the recent yellow fever epidemic. The board's president pro tem, Dr. C. A. Rice, noted in his "President's Report" to Governor Stone on November 27, 1879, that "under the present laws we stand as an advisory body only, without power to establish quarantine or law to enforce it, with no appropriations to put into operation, and none to sustain it." He further insisted that he was "duty bound to ask for further legislation to promote the efficiency and usefulness of the Board." Rice requested "wholesome legislation" in the light of the "terrible lesson we were taught in the epidemic of 1878."[8] When cities responded to the board's request, even surviving mayors included in their cities' accounts statistics of and opinions about the origin of the disease within their particular towns or communities. The majority of these officials blamed refugees infiltrating their regions as the causative agent, since the belief persisted that the contagion was portable in the form of fomites. Officials also included descriptions of preventive measures they used to curtail the spread of the contagion. As a result of this effort, the state board was able to outline the extent of yellow fever across Mississippi and provide a full picture of the disease and the breadth of its influence upon the state's citizens and economy. In other words, at one level the state board of health performed magnificently in its first real trial.

As reported in 1879, the Mississippi State Board of Health welcomed the end of the epidemic in 1878 and decided to meet that December to delineate and further hone its recommendations. At this December 10 meeting in Jackson, the state agency agreed that the "true cause of yellow fever is exotic, and that it only exists in the State by importation; that it is transportable in vessels, railroad cars, clothing, goods, etc., and that efficient quarantine regulations are competent to exclude it from the State." Absolving any local sources from blame as foci of contagion, the board outlined its reasons for requesting strong quarantine powers. The contemporary fomite theory of contagion—the belief that substances could absorb germs and subsequently be a source of contagion—obviously underpinned the group's request. The board adopted the resolution at its December meeting. This group had urged Governor Stone to call a special session of the Mississippi legislature "to amend the health laws and to enable the health authorities to guard more effectively against epidemic diseases."[9] However, these issues would not be addressed by the Mississippi legislature in 1878 and would only be vigorously discussed in 1879.

Reflecting most contemporary physicians' belief that yellow fever "poison" could survive through mild winter weather, the board also recommended in 1879 that local health boards, authorities in towns that had been infected during the past season, and the heads of all families in infected districts "overhaul ventilation in all rooms, closets, cellars, etc., in an atmosphere below the freezing point" and implement a thorough system of sanitary measures, including drainage and cleanliness. Finally, the board established twenty-six rules that outlined such recommendations as better privy construction, sewer drain regulations, and garbage disposal for local health boards to adopt in an effort to maintain better health standards in Mississippi to avoid future epidemics.[10] The state board was moving forward. Even though it lacked legislative power, its recommendations regarding cleanliness would be helpful, because its sanitary regimen would attack *A. aegypti*'s habitat. The board also displayed concern about its role in future epidemics. Rice realized all too well that even with sympathies running high, Governor Stone was unable to offer monetary assistance through the state government, "as there was no power vested in him to take State money and apply it in any way not fully authorized by law." Rice and the state board therefore resolved to create an outline of recommended initiatives for better health care and more effective methods of quarantine, such as camps with tents, food, and medical personnel, to combat future epidemics.[11] These initiatives established a willingness to engage in the sanitary revolution that would move into full swing in the last twenty years of the twentieth century.

The state board included in its recommendations and resolutions a memorial to the four board members who had died in the epidemic, Drs. W. M. Compton, E. W. Hughes, P. F. Whitehead, and A. H. Cage. Labeling their deaths "heroic," as each of the men had died while ministering to stricken Mississippians in his respective hometown, the memorial stated that these "cherished members of the Board have passed to the spirit land and peacefully rest from their labors." With this, the state board of health concluded its meeting.[12]

Even though the state board had outlined specific health needs and recommendations in 1878 in its official resolution to Governor Stone, it was not able to accomplish these goals. After the board adjourned in Jackson, all of the recommendations and resolutions were bound into an official report. Unfortunately, this report was the only result of the board's meeting. Regardless of the fact that this report reveals a concerned organization, the board was unable to accomplish all that it desired to help Mississippians. The economic atmosphere in the state at the time eclipsed the needs of its citizens for health care. Therefore, no legislative changes resulted in 1878. The U.S. Congress created the National Board of Health in March 1879, with limited powers to act more or less as a collection agency for medical statistics. The National Board of Health was further empowered in June 1879 to distribute monetary support to state and municipal health boards where aid was needed and to assume quarantine powers. The Mississippi State Board of Health hoped to take a more aggressive stance during epidemics under the guidance of this new national board. However, the U.S. Congress did not continue funding for the National Board of Health, because of a decrease in yellow fever epidemics and strife with state boards; it expired in 1883.[13]

As physicians conjectured in professional forums about yellow fever's etiology and best treatment, the Mississippi State Board of Health's cumulative statistics regarding the epidemic led to a truer picture of the effects of this visitation. For example, along the Mississippi River in Warren County, Vicksburg had been the first municipality to be infected and was the most populous city in the state at the time. In 1870, Vicksburg's records indicate a total population of 12,443; in 1880 that population was 11,814. The city's African American population in 1870 was 6,805, and whites numbered 5,638.[14] Officials recorded a few cases persisting in Vicksburg and the surrounding countryside in early November, even though the epidemic was virtually over. On November 21 health officers finally recorded the city's last yellow fever death. Vicksburg officials recorded the highest mortality figures in Mississippi's 1878 yellow fever epidemic as a result of that city's greater populace—a case number of approximately 5,000 with 872 deaths, a 17 percent death rate. The percentage of African-American deaths in Vicksburg was approximately 12 percent, with approximately 2,000 reported cases resulting in 231 deaths.[15]

In Jackson, more centrally located in the state, yellow fever cases and deaths continued to be recorded during these months. From November 2 to November 28, health workers listed nineteen yellow fever deaths. By the end of November, however, the epidemic finally ended for the city. Even though Jackson's officials claimed that quarantine restrictions had delayed yellow fever's appearance in that city until September, the disease ultimately reaped its harvest. Jackson in 1870 reported a total population of 4,234, with 2,270 whites and 1,964 African Americans.[16] After the epidemic, officials reported a total of 480 yellow fever cases, with 86 of those resulting in death, or an approximate 18 percent death rate. Even with a smaller population and fewer cases and deaths reported, the mortality rate was greater than in the larger city of Vicksburg. One difference in Jackson that was not reported consistently in other Mississippi locales was the ratio of white to black deaths. Those mortality figures were almost even, with 46 reported white deaths and 40 black deaths. However, the population percentages of the state were not even at that time. In 1878 the approximate percentages for the races were 42 percent white and 58 percent non-white. Those figures are based on the fact that in 1880 there were 479,398 whites and 652,199 non-whites recorded in the state.[17]

Although Vicksburg and Jackson reported some of the highest levels of infection and mortality in November, the epidemic ended elsewhere. At Friar's Point in Coahoma County, officials reported the last of twenty-five recorded cases on November 1. In Madison County, Canton health volunteers recorded the final case in December. Along the coast, health officials in Bay St. Louis also listed its last case in December, out of a total 690 cases. Further east, Pass Christian's officials affirmed that locale's last yellow fever death on November 22. Also on the coast, Mississippi City concluded its death count on November 14, although a nonfatal case appeared on December 10. The final yellow fever death in Biloxi occurred on November 23, in a city that suffered forty-five deaths in the course of the epidemic. Ocean Springs, across the Bay of Biloxi, listed a yellow fever death on December 5. The last coastal death occurred in Handsboro on December 24. Further north, in the small Washington County community of Leota Landing, there was only one yellow fever case, on November 21, and the victim died the next day.[18] Other locations in the hinterlands of Mississippi reported yellow fever in November and December in dwindling numbers.[19]

For a listing of the total 1878 yellow fever cases and deaths reported to the Mississippi State Board of Health, see table 2. Analysis of the data in this table explains two interesting points. First, the case/mortality ratio was higher in locales on a railroad line than in those not so situated. For example, towns such as Canton, Crystal Springs, Jackson, Lake, Lebanon, Meridian, and Water Valley recorded higher case/mortality ratios. All of those towns were located on one or the other of the two main railroad lines that had been in existence since before 1860, one running north-south and the other east-west. By contrast, locales such as Yazoo City and Benton did not experience major railroad construction until after the 1878 epidemic, and their case/mortality ratios were lower than those for communities on the main trunk lines. The Delta region also did not have extensive railroad service, and except for towns in that region on the Mississippi River, such as Greenville and Friar's Point, that area experienced fewer yellow fever cases and deaths. Second, like those locales on or near railroad lines, communities along maritime routes edging the coast, such as Bay St. Louis, Biloxi, Handsboro, Mississippi City, Ocean Springs, Pascagoula, Pass Christian, and Scranton, reported higher case/mortality ratios. All of these towns are also situated on a railroad line running between New Orleans and Mobile. Therefore, coastal communities had two inroads for the introduction of contagion. Municipalities along the Mississippi River, such as Vicksburg and Port Gibson, also recorded high numbers of yellow fever cases and deaths because of their river connection to travel and commerce. And, of course, Vicksburg confirmed the most cases and deaths, both because of its location on the Mississippi and because it was the epicenter of the epidemic. It appears then that towns on rail lines and waterways were where the most reported cases and deaths occurred, as the mechanisms of transmission are essentially the same. However, communities in the extreme southwestern corner of Mississippi, such as Natchez and Woodville, reported no cases or deaths in the epidemic, despite their location on or close proximity to the Mississippi River. The strict shotgun quarantines established there helped protect those cities, but more than likely luck had much to do with it, as these two cities had experienced yellow fever outbreaks in 1853 and other years.

Even as the epidemic waned in communities across Mississippi, the need for aid continued. Answering the call, numerous charitable organizations continued to donate generously in the last two months of the epidemic. Provisions and monetary aid flowed into Mississippi from many northern points. As Edward Blum discusses, southerners were unable to combat the disease effectively themselves in the early months of the epidemic, as supplies, personnel, and commerce quickly became exhausted or scarce. As a result, those living in the South cooperated in unprecedented ways with northerners who just thirteen years ago were considered mortal enemies.[20] Even Jefferson Davis, who had led the Confederacy in the Civil War and had been imprisoned because of his role in the conflict, composed a letter of thanks to all northerners who had generously donated funds to the stricken South. Heartbroken after the loss of his son to yellow fever, he wrote that the suffering was above and beyond that experienced in any previous epidemic. Praising the charitable contributions from the North particularly, he wrote that "The noble generosity of the Northern people in this day of our extreme affliction has been felt with deep gratitude and has done more for the fraternization of" the North and South "than many volumes of rhetorical assurance."[21]

Without a doubt, Mississippians deeply appreciated relief aid. J. L. Power, an Irishman who settled in the state, spearheaded the massive relief effort in 1878. Editor of the *Jackson Daily News* prior to the Civil War, Power had also served as the state printer in 1875; therefore, he was well qualified to undertake this huge task. Moreover, his journalistic expertise was useful as he recorded and analyzed the yellow fever epidemic and relief disbursements. In December he embarked on a statewide tour to collect yellow fever statistics and to continue making relief payments to the few remaining citizens in yellow fever zones. Power also collected letters of appreciation from Mississippians who were beneficiaries of the relief network. This correspondence reveals a genuine sense of thankfulness for received aid and expresses sincere gratitude to the donors. For instance, on December 10 a citizen from Osyka wrote that "it would be impossible to tell you

Table 2. Reported yellow fever cases and deaths in Mississippi in 1878

Locales	Total Cases	Total Deaths
Bay St. Louis	690	82
Benton	3	1
Biloxi	295	45
Bolton	144	34
Bovina	20	7
Brown's Plantations (Hinds County)	21	4
Byram	10	1
Canton and Vicinity	924	180
Carrollton	200	5
Claiborne County	600	150
Crystal Springs	112	44
Dry Grove, Lebanon Church	125	52
Duck Hill and Vicinity	—	11
Friar's Point	25	7
Gainesville (Hancock County)	5	2
Garner's Station	7	—
Goodrich Landing (Mississippi River)	—	12
Greenville	903	301
Grenada and Vicinity	1040	326
Horn Lake	2	2
Handsboro	200	69
Hernando	240	80
Holly Springs	1239	309
Iuka	6	3
Jackson	480	86
Lake	300	86
Lebanon (Hinds County)	90	10
Leota Landing	1	1
Livingston (Madison County)	15	10
McComb City	63	21
Meridian	400	91
Mississippi City	200	15
Moscow	71	35
Ocean Springs	175	30
Okolona	300	45
Pascagoula	8	3
Pass Christian	199	23
Pearlington	201	24
Port Gibson	620	115

Continued on the next page

Table 2. (*continued*)

Locales	Total Cases	Total Deaths
Refuge Landing (Washington County)	19	11
Rocky Springs (Claiborne County)	—	38
Scranton	60	20
Smith's Station (Hinds County)	16	—
Stoneville	23	15
Spring Hill	15	6
Sulphur Springs (Madison County)	15	5
Summit	5	2
Senatobia	26	7
Tallulah	25	5
Terrene and Vicinity (Bolivar County)	12	4
Terry	20	—
Tunica	—	5
Vicksburg	5000	1149
Vicinity of Vicksburg	900	300
Water Valley	200	64
Winterville	20	3
Winona	—	3
Winterville and vicinity (Washington County)	151	26
Yazoo City	17	9
Total Reports: 60	**Total Cases: 16,461**	**Total Deaths: 4118**

Sources: *Conclusions of the Board of Experts Authorized by Congress to Investigate the Yellow Fever Epidemic of 1878;* and Spinzig, *Yellow Fever.* Both of these sources list individual localities and their yellow fever cases and deaths. Between the two sources, however, there were some discrepancies, usually amounting to just a few cases or deaths. In instances where there was a discrepancy, the higher number was listed in the table.

what relief the money you gave me was to us. God alone knows what would have become of us but for your timely visit. What you gave me was the only money we have had this summer. . . . I pray God may forever bless you and yours. He will surely watch over one who had lightened so many sinking hearts." In Water Valley, a woman and her three children also received money from the Masons, and she explained that "her tearful thanks fully attested her deep obligations and the timely aid it gave her and her three babes." F. M. Featherstun of Vicksburg, the minister who had lost almost his entire family to yellow fever, expressed his gratitude for monetary relief when he wrote that "amid sore bereavements, my happy home now desolate and deserted, I thank God that He has given me precious and honored friends, whose tender kindnesses do so much to soothe the wounded spirit. May the Lord bless you in soul and preserve your useful life." These sincere expressions of gratitude reveal the feelings of many less-articulate Mississippians and illustrate the success of the massive relief efforts in 1878.[22]

Total monetary aid to Mississippi was substantial. The state received $522,632.42 from sources such as Masonic lodges, Sunday school collections, private donations, and fund-raising events across the country. This amount, however, does not include any allowance for material goods from the U.S. government or donations of disinfectants or free transportation provided for physicians and nurses traveling to and within Mississippi by railroad. The generosity exhibited by all states in the nation was significant and helped to heal the psyche of a nation recently torn apart by civil war and Reconstruction.[23]

For an account of total relief aid sent to Mississippi in 1878, see table 3. As the table shows, Mississippians received generous amounts of aid; in fact, Vicksburg received the staggering amount of $263,045. Power records that this sum derived from several sources, including the Howard Association ($184,000), the city of Vicksburg ($10,000), and the "Masons, Odd Fellows, Hebrews, Knights of Pythias, Hibernians, and Religious Bodies" ($47,000). Vicksburg was by far the city hit hardest in the epidemic, and it received the most financial assistance. Masons from across the United States, including Arizona Territory, California, Dakota Territory, New York (with the largest collection of $12,952.68), and the Sandwich Islands ($82.75), collected money for yellow fever relief. Even Masons in Tennessee, who were struggling with their own epidemic in Memphis, contributed $21.[24]

Mississippians also participated in the monetary relief effort. For example, G. T. McGehee from Woodville gave $13 from an anonymous donor to Power for the effort, explaining that the money was from a female acquaintance of his and that it was "the result of a mite collection taken up by her, to be disposed of as your judgment may dictate." He further added that "sincere expressions of heartfelt sympathy" were included in his letter for "our afflicted friends in Jackson[.] We pray for their speedy deliverance."[25] In the light of all the aid, the state government's failure to provide relief—or even help with distribution—was even more evident. Dr. Rice of the Mississippi State Board of Health praised the "munificent donations from our Northern brethren and from the Masons, Odd Fellows, and other benevolent and charitable societies and institutions," but he chastised Mississippi officials, because "it was apparent to all that Mississippi, in the capacity of a state, was doing nothing to supply the wants or to ameliorate the suffering of their stricken people."[26] The criticism did not apply to individual

Mississippians, however. Although their resources were either stretched to the maximum or virtually nonexistent as a result of the economic hardships resulting from the epidemic, intrastate cooperation and compassion was evident.

Support for Mississippi and other parts of the South was not limited to money or commodities. Ordinary people throughout the country provided spiritual support for the stricken regions through numerous organized religious services and other public functions. For example, President Rutherford B. Hayes declared November 28, 1878, the national day of annual Thanksgiving when Americans recognized their blessings. However, that year some officials included an acknowledgment of the yellow fever epidemic. Governors in various states addressed the epidemic in their Proclamations of Thanksgiving. Even though Thanksgiving Day was supposed to be observed in recognition of the bounty of the land and blessings of the country, several governors offered condolences to and support for the South in their Thanksgiving Day proclamations. For instance, Texas governor R. B. Hubbard announced that the United States had been fortunate to be in a time of peace "at home and abroad" and that all citizens, in view of the recent yellow fever outbreak, should invoke the "mercies of God upon the orphan and the widow, the poor and the desolate, of those stricken States" and "we should, as a people, render thanks to Almighty God for the renewed evidence which these calamities have given that the American people are still one people in all the elements of Christian charity, brotherhood, and union." New Jersey's governor, former Union general George B. McClellan, proclaimed that his state's citizens had been "mercifully . . . shielded against the pestilence which has wrought such havoc among our brethren of other States, and we have good cause to thank Him, in their behalf, that the course of the seasons has been interrupted in order to bring their terrible trials to a close." He further outlined the continued need of "fellow-citizens—once arrayed in arms against us, but now, through God's mercy, happily reunited with us—" to provide "relief and aid beyond the power of their immediate neighbors to afford." McClellan suggested that citizens in New Jersey could collect money at their Thanksgiving Day church services for what he called a "thank-offering" for the "relief of our unfortunate fellow-citizens of the afflicted districts of the South." In fact, the majority of McClellan's one-page proclamation addressed the stricken South.[27] Illinois governor Shelby M. Cullom requested that citizens in his state give thanks to "the Divine favor" that yellow fever had not appeared in their state and that they had been spared the "ravages of the pestilence" that had afflicted other regions. Throughout the United States, citizens who observed Thanksgiving Day in 1878 remembered the yellow fever victims in the South and doubtless breathed sighs of relief that they had not been affected by the disease.[28]

Table 3. Relief aid received in Mississippi locales in 1878

City/Locale	Masons and Odd Fellow Aid	Other Aid
Bolton	$1637.00	
Brandon	$50.00	
Byram	$50.00	
Canton	$1355.00	$22,238.57
Crystal Springs	$50.00	
Dry Grove	$2565.60	
Edwards	$450.00	
Garner	$800.00	
Greenville	$5082.40	$31,068.66
Grenada	$8790.00	$24,493.43
Hernando	$500.00	$3242.20
Holly Springs	$8790.00	$54,859.42
Jackson	$2854.65	$17,617.07
Lake	$2875.00	$4225.00
Lawrence Station	$50.00	
Lebanon neighborhood	$202.00	
Macon	$500.00	
Meridian	$13,631.55	
McComb City	$1781.55	
Near Baldwin's Ferry	$50.00	
Oakland	$300.00	
Osyka	$861.00	
Port Gibson	$3250.00	$20,678.27
Senatobia	$250.00	
Sharon	$150.00	
Summit	$25.00	
Tallahatchie County	$850.00	
Tchula	$110.00	
Terry	$50.00	
Tillatoba	$500.00	
Vicksburg	$13,045.70	$250,000.00
Water Valley	$3307.93	$5578.82
Winona	$30.00	
Miscellaneous	$319.35	
Total	**$75,099.13**	

Continued on the next page

Table 3. (*continued*)

City/Locale	Masons and Odd Fellow Aid	Other Aid
Total cash contributions to Bolton, Edwards, Osyka, McComb City, Dry Grove, Yazoo City, Garner, Oakland, Tallahatchie County, Senatobia, and other places		$35,000.00
Cash contributed by Power, not included in above acknowledgments		$50,000.00
Total cash received in Mississippi for relief		$522,632.42
Estimated value of United States' supplies, medicines, etc., and freight and travel charges		$150,000.00

Source: Power, *The Epidemic of 1878.*

This outpouring of monetary aid and prayer from people outside the state was significant. McClellan referred to "fellow-citizens" in his Thanksgiving remembrance and expressed relief that the South and the North were reunited. This expression and others like it certainly do not seem concerned with or alarmed at the new Democratic regime in Mississippi. In fact, the generous aid to the state does not hint at any dissatisfaction regarding the state's political makeup. With the Compromise of 1877, when Congress withdrew the last federal troops from South Carolina, Florida, and Louisiana and reestablished home rule in the South, Republicans in a compromise with the Democrats assured Rutherford B. Hayes the presidency in exchange for the end of Reconstruction. With that compromise, the nation abandoned African Americans to their fate and politicians basically closeted the "bloody shirt" of sectionalism and racism until the 1880s.

Just as Mississippians accepted outside relief and thoughtful prayers for the most part, they were also deeply thankful for help from within. Mississippians poured forth letters of thanks to the various intrastate relief agencies as well as outside aid groups. In addition to individual letters of appreciation, newspapers throughout the state published tributes to those agencies that had helped so diligently in the epidemic, particularly highlighting J. L. Power's efforts. These accolades reveal that Mississippians were grateful to have received generous donations through and from the Masons and Odd Fellows and that they appreciated Power's organization and distribution of these gifts. For example, Dr. C. A. Rice of Vicksburg, president of the state board of health, acknowledged the generous relief donations when he reported to Governor Stone that the "munificent donations from our Northern brethren and from the Masons, Odd Fellows, and other benevolent and charitable societies and institutions" were like "one grand and mighty stream of charity and love fed with its thousand fountains of affection."[29] In Water Valley and other places across the state, Power prudently distributed money to the destitute, orphans, and widows in the districts visited by the epidemic. According to the *Water Valley Courier*, he consulted with leading citizens and officers of the state's Masonic and Odd Fellows lodges before he distributed funds to those most in need. When he traveled to Holly Springs, the *Holly Springs Reporter* wrote of his visit to that town and stated that he was "looking after the destitute, rendering them relief, and gathering facts connected with the plague, for use in the history of the pestilence which he is preparing." His noble work did not cease even when the epidemic began to abate. Mississippians were reminded in the *Water Valley Courier* that "the kindly spirit in which these funds were donated to our suffering, sick and dying ones, should and does warm all hearts with deepest gratitude and make us all feel more kindly of our common humanity than we have ever done before."[30]

The flood of financial, material, and spiritual aid during the epidemic overshadowed, if only for a brief time, national antagonisms. Many sentiments were expressed regarding the healing of the nation's psyche. Relief aid was often emblematic of a national spirit that could emerge to encompass regions once bitterly opposed to each other, regardless of some reticence. Thomas S. Gathright of College Station, Texas, wrote that relief efforts are lessons illustrating that "when our people come to understand each other a strong bond of sympathy and fraternity is found to hold them together . . . so that all sections of our Union may serve as mutually protecting braces."[31]

Gathright's assessment of the charitable organizations operating during the epidemic surfaces as the heart of Mississippi's response to the epidemic. A strong sense of self-reliance carried people through the tough times. As a result, during the epidemic communities took care of their own yellow fever victims, albeit often with charitable donations from either within or outside Mississippi. Citizens were able to direct the outflow of assistance and thus retain their self-reliance and sense of honor. This spirit of self-help would shortly form the basis of a public health movement supported by outside money. However, racial considerations did affect who received aid. In 1878 there was no oversight committee to ensure the equitable distribution of aid during the peak months of activity to the end of the year. Communities still relied on their own to distribute aid equitably in the late stages of the epidemic.

Even though relief disbursements through November and December did not rival the previous months' totals, contributions to the destitute were still impressive. In those months, contributors donated $10,566.87 to Mississippians who had been affected by the epidemic. The majority of the disbursements in November and December went to orphans and to widows with children. For example, W. M. Thornton of Lake received $250 on behalf of the children left parentless from the Lowry, Davison, and Crouch families. In Grenada, fifty-one orphans and ten widows received $1,825 to help relieve their dire situations. The disbursements through these last two months helped to provide for those who were unable to care for themselves.[32]

As relief payments continued in November and December, businesses began operations to satisfy customers who for months had been without all types of consumer goods. Local health boards convened throughout Mississippi in early November to lift quarantine restrictions so that businesses could restore commerce to the state's citizens. Jackson County officials called a special meeting on November 8 for the purpose of "raising all quarantine restrictions." The quarantine officer there reported that he had "smashed all his fumigation pots and washed sulphur from his hands," since his services were no longer required. The local health board also claimed that "although communication by rail and water has been opened up, it will yet be two weeks before people generally visit the cities so recently infected by the dreadful yellow disease, as they do not feel perfectly secure in going into those places so soon." Regardless, the board was optimistic that "business will begin to open up, and in a short time, trade and commerce will again be active."[33] In Brookhaven, merchants reported that they had received "large and splendid stocks" to "furnish the people with everything they need" as they returned to their homes.[34] Yazoo City officials arranged for quarantine restrictions to be lifted and expected commerce to return to normal quickly as refugees returned home. By November 8, several frosts had occurred in the Yazoo City region, so its citizens were more willing to come back. Yazoo City officials predicted: "We may reasonably expect that our streets will soon be crowded with the fleecy staple [cotton], and our city present that stir and animation as in other days."[35] Desiring the restoration of civic and personal normality, citizens in Greenville reported that their city streets were once again "thronged with people" and that all activities were finally being revived. Along the coast, sawmills in Handsboro and Moss Point resumed operations as mill owners and employees journeyed back to their homes. After months of stagnant business, Mississippi was finally able to begin economic recovery. Health officials in Jackson County offered an entreaty on November 8 that "God grant we may never have another such season of disease, death and destruction."[36] That supplication must have been the sentiment of all Mississippians who returned to their homes and communities in November and December.

Returning refugees poured into Vicksburg with every incoming boat and train. As a major port of entry on the Mississippi River, the city witnessed a steady stream of citizens returning through its terminals and ports. "Hearty greetings" welcomed the "tearful and weary" pilgrims. Local retailers such as Leis, Brothers and Company and H. Drucker and Company had reopened in order to provide necessities to those returning citizens. The city most devastated in the recent epidemic could also cease mourning and revert to optimism.[37]

Throughout the summer of 1878, Mississippians had experienced chilling consequences of the yellow fever epidemic. In November, however, the state's citizens were finally able to hope as the case numbers and deaths drastically declined. For a horror-filled six months, the nation transcended its sectional problems and joined together to console the plague-ridden South as outpourings of aid soothed old battle wounds. By December the South began to recover economically from the devastating effects of the yellow fever epidemic. Mississippians were returning to their homes in droves, rebuilding their lives and the livelihood of their towns and state. The 1878 yellow fever epidemic was over.

8
Conclusion

O year to be remembered for its woe!
—Ellen F. Hebron, "The Physicians of 1878"

The 1878 yellow fever epidemic was paradoxical. It brought much suffering and disruption, but it also brought a sense of restored order to Mississippi. Where there was success, it could be credited to traditional values. Where there was death, the victims were sometimes lauded as representatives of a glorious past. Government failed to help, but Democrats remained ascendant. As citizens resumed their daily lives there was a sense that something was finally right again in "redeemed" Mississippi, despite the presence of so much that was patently wrong.

Although it lacked empowerment both legislatively and monetarily, the Mississippi State Board of Health continued to coordinate community relief efforts by issuing disinfection recommendations, collecting data, and suggesting quarantines. Under the circumstances, the board did a commendable job in an extremely difficult situation. According to its records, the last official yellow fever death in Mississippi was on November 28 in Jackson. The board officially ended the epidemic on that date, although isolated cases continued to appear. Across the nation, local health officials and state health boards in approximately two hundred stricken communities collated information regarding the epidemic. By some accounts, the total number of recorded cases in the United States was 69,187, with 16,296 deaths (a 23.5 percent death rate). New Orleans alone had seen 4,046 deaths, and Memphis recorded between 5,000 and 6,000.[1] Because of faulty record keeping, hesitancy in recognizing yellow fever, and poor communication, precise numbers are difficult to establish, as illustrated by the discrepancies between these numbers and those in table 4. Mississippi reported 4,100 deaths out of an approximate state population of 970,000, more than 25 percent of the total deaths nationwide. Within the state, at least 4.2 percent of the population died in the epidemic, including fifty physicians and four members of the Mississippi State Board of Health. Ordinary citizens buried family and friends in record numbers. As Dr. Gant stated, "the epidemic of 1878 should go down in history as the most malignant, widespread and fatal that ever visited the United States" (see table 4).[2] In Louisiana, Mississippi, Tennessee, Alabama, Florida, Arkansas, Kentucky, and Missouri, yellow fever cases totaled 51,553, with Tennessee, Louisiana, and Mississippi accounting for the vast majority (50,489). Most of the recorded deaths also occurred in these three states: 11,719 out of a 12,063 southern total. Non-southern states recorded only 101 deaths. The average mortality rate for the South was 32.8 percent, while the two northern states, Illinois and Ohio, had a mortality rate of 55.3 percent.

As the epidemic faded in Mississippi, newspapers across the state began to demand a national organization to help administer quarantines and assist with relief. For six months Mississippians had labored under the effects of an epidemic with virtually no state government aid, and many in the state believed it was now time to look to the federal government for help. Realizing that the state was woefully underprepared for an extensive epidemic, newspaper editors addressed the pressing issues of organized governmental relief efforts and uniform quarantine laws and enforcement. On December 12, 1878, the editors of the *Crystal Springs Monitor* summed up the state's overriding perspective: "the fearful spread of this pestilence has awakened a very general public sentiment in favor of national sanitary administration," including quarantine control and the supervision of inter- and intrastate commerce during epidemics. Economic advantages associated with government control in time of crisis probably spurred the opinions of the editors, for they stated that the national board should have an advisory role only, except to help state and local governments enforce quarantine laws.[3]

The federal government did, however, react to and become engaged in the relief efforts to the South during the epidemic. The Yellow Fever National Relief Commission, organized on September 11, 1878, to address the epidemic—the agency that sponsored the expedition of the *John M. Chambers*—met in Washington, D.C., regularly to consider plans for future actions to help in the crisis.[4] The commission made public the receipts and accounts of disbursements of the funds that were channeled through it. Even with this organization, the many requests for monetary and provisional aid continued to tax its resources and to overwhelm administrative efforts. Therefore, it joined the ranks calling for a federal regulatory body. To understand the myriad problems better, the commission then created a special investigatory team, headed by Dr. John M. Woodworth, supervising surgeon general of the U.S. Marine Hospital Service, to gather and compile statistics from fever-stricken regions. Woodworth was to present a report later that fall.

Difficulties arose, however, in efforts to create a federal agency. In September 1878 a clash developed between personnel of the leading medical agencies. An intense rivalry between Woodworth and Dr. John Shaw Billings, vice-president

Table 4. Yellow Fever Cases and Deaths in the United States during the 1878 epidemic

Locales	Cases	Deaths	Mortality Rates
Louisiana	24,068	4903	20.3%
Mississippi	12,703	3277	25.7%
Tennessee	13,718	3539	25.7%
Alabama	501	129	25.7%
Florida	40	19	47.5%
Arkansas	112	9	8.0%
Kentucky	336	135	40.1%
Missouri	75	52	69.3%
Illinois	94	47	50.0%
Ohio	89	54	60.6%
Total	**51737**	**12,164**	**23.5%**

Source: Spinzig, *Yellow Fever,* 173. Discrepancies result because of home burials, inaccurate records, and mistaken diagnoses. Regardless of statistical choices, the number of yellow fever casualties was significant.

of the American Public Health Association (APHA), further hindered the already difficult task. Both men were able physicians who had served with distinction in the Civil War and had become prominent figures in the medical profession. The conflict arose when widespread support for a federal health agency, capable of regulating quarantines and enforcing medical standards, developed during the epidemic. Each man coveted the position as chief health officer for such an agency, and each had loyal supporters grounded in diverse agendas.[5] When Woodworth organized the Yellow Fever Commission as a fact-finding entity, he sparked contention, since Billings now regarded him as a rival. Under the agenda of the newly created commission, Woodworth and his special team of investigators were to conclude and submit their report by November 19, after the epidemic receded.

In November the APHA convened in Richmond to discuss the public health issue and to hear what Woodworth's special commission had to report. Because the commission had had so little time to gather information, Woodworth's first report to the APHA was sketchy and only reiterated what was already known. The commission had made hurried visits to New Orleans, Baton Rouge, Vicksburg, Port Gibson, and Grenada to gather statistics, but because of time constraints, an incomplete accounting resulted. In addition, Woodworth apparently overstepped his authority by scheduling meetings at the Richmond convention to discuss various aspects of the investigation. When others criticized him for exceeding his authority in this way, he replied that he felt "very much hurt" by the criticism.[6]

Because of the inadequacy of Woodworth's findings, the National Relief Commission was sharply criticized. Woodworth expressed concern over this disapproval, since he had been the director of the special investigatory team. Apparently, complaints about the report's inconclusiveness surfaced after Billings pointed out the problems to Woodworth. Billings, however, was not the only critic of Woodworth's work. Major William T. Walthall of Mobile, a volunteer in Memphis during the epidemic, also complained that the reports were a "waste of two days' valuable time with inconsequential tedium."[7] Woodworth's reputation appeared compromised as a result.

The problems at the Richmond meeting, however, were not centered on the commission's inadequate findings or on the rivalry between the two men. The real crux of the problem was the matter of states' rights. The APHA asserted that both quarantines and expanded sanitation efforts would control yellow fever and that both were to be regulated under state control with a strong medical community influence. Many believed that a national board should only have advisory power to help local and state governments enforce quarantines, and that any expansion of those powers would infringe upon the efforts of states to exert authority within their own borders regarding other aspects of health control. Although Billings desired the position as chief medical officer on a federally created board, the APHA wanted to keep health care apolitical and under the auspices of medical personnel. The core of the conflict was best summed up in a resolution made at the APHA meeting at Richmond: "That, in the deliberate judgment of this association, it is the duty of every State to establish and adequately maintain an efficient state board of health, and to as great an extent as practicable contribute to the protection of the public health within its own commonwealth, and to that of the whole country; that the power and duties of the state boards of health should be so well defined by law and so fully provided for in the polity of state administration, that the sanitary interests and protection of all places in the state shall be insured."[8] This affirmation of states' rights resonated strongly throughout the South and the rest of the nation in the postwar atmosphere. But Billings and his supporters also had clear evidence that southern states—especially Mississippi—lacked the resources and political will to take care of their own. In the end, the South itself took the initiative in favor of a national organization.

President Rutherford Hayes, in his annual message to the Forty-fifth Congress, asked that body to give its attention to the quarantine issue, as the South had suffered terribly in the recent epidemic. Therefore, on December 2, three senators representing the states most affected by the recent epidemic—Isham G.

Harris of Tennessee, James B. Eustis of Louisiana, and Lucius Q. C. Lamar of Mississippi—presented resolutions calling for national health legislation. Lamar drafted Senate Resolution 1462, which called for a national bureau of public health. Lamar has been aptly described as an "industrial-commercial" Democrat who identified more with commercial interests than with agrarian concerns.[9] Mississippians with the same vision as Lamar were building a framework upon which to construct a New South—a region with industrial development and a diverse economy connected to northern industrialists. Health care needed to be part of this vision, because only a healthy population can make an economy thrive. In the twentieth century this notion would be a key factor behind public health development in Mississippi as the state fought its reputation as an unhealthy region.[10] Therefore, when Lamar outlined a national health board, he was envisioning Mississippi in a new light—involved in national agendas. However, because the APHA did not want a strong federal agency, debate ensued in Congress regarding which agency could best prevent and explain the disease.[11]

After extensive consultation and investigation, the Board of Experts reported its findings to Congress on January 30, 1879. This board's composition and role reflected compromises between the Senate and the House of Representatives, and it was directed to further investigate the yellow fever epidemic. It consisted of eleven physicians and one civil engineer. The board recommended strict quarantines as the best tool to prevent future epidemics and concluded that the disease had been imported into the United States. A bill introduced by Representative Jonas H. McGowan of Michigan (H.R. 6500) outlined a health commission consisting of nine members who would be under the oversight of the Treasury Department. No representation from the U.S. Marine Hospital Service would be included in its membership; therefore, Woodworth was excluded at the outset. After much wrangling, the McGowan Bill, or Public Health Association Bill, was signed into law by President Hayes on March 3, 1879. The National Board of Health would be mostly an advisory entity, and as John H. Ellis explains, "Its limited functions were restricted to investigation of matters relating to public health, an advisory relation to federal departments and state governments, and responsibility for reporting to Congress a plan for national health administration."[12] The southern Democrats who had allied themselves with Woodworth against the APHA now found themselves backing the losing faction.[13]

Additional legislation soon helped the South with quarantine problems. On June 2, 1879, Congress expanded the powers of the National Board of Health to include a federal quarantine law when states were unable to protect their citizens and to provide monetary support to state and municipal health boards. The Mississippians who had first backed such a plan had reason to be satisfied now.

Congress stipulated that the national board would exist for only four years unless further appropriations were made. The national board went into effect just as the new yellow fever season was beginning. Regardless of its shortcomings and potentially brief existence, the National Board of Health could now enact, to some degree, legislation concerning yellow fever and other infectious diseases and could establish a national quarantine law.[14] The board quickly established a four-pronged plan to deal with yellow fever: quarantine procedures, federal inspectors, federal monetary aid, and specific quarantine locations.[15] During future epidemics, federal quarantine laws would restrict traffic and travel across the South.

The Mississippi State Board of Health endorsed the new federal health board on July 15. At the state board's annual meeting in Jackson, members voted to "adopt [the] rules and regulations of the National Board of Health as proposed for the government of State and municipal Boards of Health." They also fine-tuned their quarantine plan for the 1879 yellow fever season by establishing six quarantine points—two against New Orleans and four against Memphis. All of these stations were located either on railroad lines or the Mississippi River. As Wirt Johnston, secretary of the state board, observed, Mississippi now had "harmony and concert of action" to keep the dreaded scourge from the state.[16] With these coordinated efforts between state and county boards, Mississippi officials created an infrastructure that began with actions against yellow fever but would ultimately lead to a vital public health system.

Problems centered on a National Board of Health were not the only considerations for Mississippians. The state's economy had been adversely affected by the epidemic at a time when Mississippi definitely could not endure too many more economic downturns—the 1860s and 1870s had been stressful enough. Yet the state had experienced an estimated $40,000,000 loss as a result of the epidemic.[17] Industries that depended on interstate commerce, such as railroads, were hit particularly hard by commercial interruptions. Bradley Bond maintains that railroads were "agents of New South economic expansion," but with sustained losses during the epidemic, railroads and associated commercial enterprises had been heavy losers.[18] Most railroad lines could not contribute to the economic recovery of the South during the epidemic because they were shut down by quarantine restrictions; only one line remained active throughout the epidemic. That line, the Chicago, St. Louis, and New Orleans Railroad, ran through the heartland of Mississippi. Local quarantines for this line began on August 1 and continued until October 25; however, the railroad maintained operations to relieve fever-stricken communities along its line as much it could. After the epidemic, the company detailed its losses:

Decrease in earnings from August 1 to November 1	$311,500.00
Numbers of pounds of freight carried free	8,049,946
Number of passengers carried free	1,130
Money value of free transportation	$32,879.82
Number of officers and employees died of fever	79
Number of sick and recovered	158[19]

The average number of employees for the Chicago, St. Louis, and New Orleans Railroad was twenty-five hundred. During the epidemic the company hauled freight, physicians, nurses, and ordinary passengers free of charge. However, railroad employees experienced significant layoffs because of the company's charitable efforts. In August, 222 workers were laid off, while in September that number rose to 624. October showed the highest incidence, with 733. During the peak epidemic months of August, September, and October, workers for the Chicago, St. Louis, and New Orleans Railroad Company experienced a progressive jobless rate. For example, in August the percentage was 8.9 percent; in September it was 25.0 percent; and by October it peaked at 29.3 percent. The idle workers were unable to contribute substantially to the economy during the epidemic and more than likely became dependent on the charity of others.

Another rail line traversing southern Mississippi, the New Orleans and Mobile Railroad, experienced similar problems. During the epidemic months the main railroad route from New Orleans to Mobile was shut down when quarantines halted commerce and travel. In those areas along the Mississippi Gulf Coast that still offered limited railroad service, the conductors did not bother to collect fares because of citizens' lack of money and as a response to their recent hardships. The company also estimated that it hauled 150,000 pounds of freight free of charge and ran 1,550 miles of special emergency rail service, resulting in a $300,000 loss during the three major epidemic months. This loss triggered the layoff of 500 railroad employees. Of the employees who were retained by the railroad company, 145 contracted yellow fever and 71 died. To recoup some of its monetary losses, the railroad tried to sue Mobile for $80,000 per month for stopping its trains from running through that municipality. The threat did not work, and the quarantine restricted rail commerce and travel until November 3.[20] The problems of this one rail line illustrate the immense complications resulting from quarantine restrictions. Scenarios such as this one occurred throughout the affected regions.

More unusual incidents also resulted as railroad companies experienced the devastating economic effects of the 1878 epidemic. In Greenville, the Greenville Construction Company had built nine miles of railroad line from that city to Stoneville in 1877. However, railroad operations were suspended when yel-

Table 5. Cotton production in Mississippi, 1877–1879: Acreage, production, and yield

Year	Acres harvested (x 1000 acres)	Production (x 1000 bales)	Yield per harvested acre (pounds of cotton lint)
1877	1,964	803	184
1878	2,025	725	160
1879	2,102	963	208

Sources: McCandless, *Base Book,* 6; Wall, *The State of Mississippi,* 11. Wall was the commissioner for the State Board of Immigration and Agriculture.

low fever appeared in the Mississippi Delta. The Greenville line offered free trips out of the city to what was believed to be a safe haven, Stoneville. After two months of inactivity and lost revenue, the line finally resumed operations. However, when the train began its first run after its hiatus, the grass had grown so high on its tracks that when the engine rolled over the tall weeds, they caught on fire from the sparks flying out of the coal-fueled engine. As a result, two cars carrying cotton bales and another containing cotton seed burned.[21] The ensuing losses to both the railroad and the cotton growers were disastrous, as economic recovery from the epidemic was just commencing.

Another industry that experienced steep losses in Mississippi was cotton. Even though more acres were planted to cotton in 1878 than in 1877, bale production did not increase. The spring planting season in 1878 was not influenced by the epidemic; hence, the acreage cultivated was not affected, and in fact increased (see table 5). In 1877 and 1879 we see comparatively higher figures in production and yield per acre.[22] The difference between the production in 1878 and 1879 is 238,000 bales. An examination of the number of bales produced in the state between 1877 and 1879 reveals a less-than-normal per-acre yield for 1878, likely resulting from a lack of laborers, since picking and ginning cotton is done in the fall, which was also the peak yellow fever period.[23] In those regions of Mississippi where yellow fever was minimal or nonexistent, cotton production continued, but in other areas of the state that suffered effects of the epidemic, planters lost a greater percentage of that crop. Also, quarantine restrictions blocked some transportation routes and ports used by planters to haul and ship their cotton. The report of the congressional Board of Experts states that "this loss is very large, amounting to millions of dollars, but it cannot be correctly estimated."[24]

With the mass disruptions resulting from the epidemic, it is amazing that production of the crop occurred at all. Adding to this scenario, the usual capital invested by citizens in land, houses, watercraft, machinery, vehicles, implements, and commodities was lost, because health needs superseded individual purchases and investments during the epidemic. No exact monetary estimate can be made of these losses, but the impact was great as stores and supply houses remained closed for extended periods.

Health care costs related to the epidemic were far reaching and difficult to calculate. The Board of Experts prepared an estimate for the cost of caring for the sick, placing a monetary value on specific aspects:

Cost of sickness of 120,000 for 25 days at 50¢ per day	$1,500,000
Cost of medical attendance	$3,600,000
Cost of 18,000 funerals, at $20 each	$360,000
Cost of special sanitary work	$100,000
Total	$5,560,000[25]

In Mississippi and throughout the South, charitable contributions helped offset the $5,560,000. If we apply the same twenty-five-day convalescence period at a cost of 50¢ per day for Mississippi's 12,703 cases, $158,787.50 was expended for the care of Mississippians in addition to the $3,600,000 for medical attendance.[26]

Health officers in cities across Mississippi reported expenditures and crippling losses during the epidemic. For example, Dr. A. T. Semmes, president of the Madison County Board of Health, outlined Canton's economic losses in his accounting to the state board of health. Semmes reckoned that Canton, situated on the Chicago, St. Louis, and New Orleans Railroad, lost $16,500 in potential labor by calculating the value of time lost by unemployed, convalescing yellow fever patients at an average of a dollar per day. Adding the cost of medical attendance, medicines, nursing care, funerals, sanitary work, and quarantine maintenance, he reached a total of $22,000. As an added loss, he wrote that in attempting to control yellow fever, officials destroyed citizens' clothes and bedding valued at $1,000.[27] These are approximate totals, but with some sketchy reports, especially in the case of African Americans, absolute summations are impossible. However, these reports provide a picture of Mississippi's economic hardships. State officials calculated to the best of their ability the same type of losses and expenditures, indicating severe economic setbacks resulting from the epidemic.

When the yellow fever epidemic ended, some people outside Mississippi recognized racial disparity and strife as another result of the epidemic. In a few letters received after the epidemic, Governor Stone endured tirades that revealed unresolved racial hostility. During the epidemic, white officials usually controlled the distribution of monetary and provisional relief aid. Deep resentment between black and white communities arose as whites accused African Americans of receiving free handouts, and African Americans believed aid allotments to be unequal, as in Vicksburg. As a result, race relations in the state were adversely affected. Moreover, Jim Crowism was on the Democratic agenda for the near future.

Some letters to Stone reveal deep racial hatred. The governor received such a letter in September from an unidentified sender, an African American who might once have lived in Mississippi. As the fever raged in Mississippi, the writer sent the letter from Baltimore. It opened by calling Stone an "Infamous Scoundrel!" The tone of the letter was decidedly hostile and inflammatory. Stone was referred to as a "Democratic devil," an "unjust cowardly dog," and a rascal. The main point of the letter, however, was that Yellow Jack punished Mississippi for injustices heaped upon the state's African Americans: "The wrath of God is now let loose upon the South for all their wickedness. . . . Memphis is desolate, Glory to God for his avenging rod, the Solid South will soon be a Solid Wilderness and better people will go to inhabit it and all the murderous Mississippi devils will be in hell driven by Negroes whom they murdered upon the earth. . . . The Southern people are a Whiskey-drinking, Tobacco-chewing, constant-spitting, Negro-Hating, Negro-killing, red-handed, ignorant uneducated, Uncivilized set of devils."[28]

After the epidemic ended, a bitter letter arrived from Washington, D.C., apparently from the same author. This time the writer expressed disappointment that the recent bout of yellow fever had not killed all of the Mississippian "infernal hell hounds." The author continued: "The Yellow Fever failed to correct you Southern devils and so in 1880 you will all be totally annihilated and not only defeated." National elections occurred in 1880, so the author could have been referring to those when he predicted problems for the southerners that year. The closing regards were, "I remain Your master & superior[,] A. Negro."[29] Obviously, the letter writer was upset at the recent turn of political events in Mississippi. However, it would be many years before African Americans would once again be included in southern politics.

Not all the effects of the yellow fever epidemic were negative. A humanitarian relief effort surpassed all expectations, particularly in contrast to the upheaval of the Civil War and Reconstruction. The nation pulled together to relieve all those struggling regions, and Mississippians were the recipients of generous monetary relief aid. Additionally, an outpouring of devotion and care for the yellow fever victims in the form of prayers, letters, and national observances occurred across the nation. Sectional antagonism briefly fell by the wayside as northerners reached out to southerners both monetarily and spiritually.

As devastating as the 1853 epidemic had been in terms of lives lost, no yellow fever epidemic before or since the 1878 scourge has rivaled its widespread death and destruction. Mississippians had to cope with this disease as best they could. Aid and hundreds of volunteers from outside of the state bolstered plague-stricken citizens as their state organizations failed them. The tumultuous 1870s and the uncertain times during this epidemic indeed strained the state politically as leaders continued to lock out African Americans. Economically, the beleaguered state eventually overcame the effects of the epidemic. Many Mississippians had died of yellow fever even as the medical community argued about the disease's modes of transmission and treatment. In the ensuing years the state would experience other, lesser epidemics, but by 1901 the mosquito transmission theory would be proven and generally accepted in the medical community, and yellow fever would no longer pose a major threat to Mississippi and the rest of the South. The final epidemic would occur in 1905 and would demonstrate successful efforts of health officials to control the mosquito vector. Expanded medical knowledge explaining the etiology of yellow fever, combined with prompt and effective precautionary actions taken by state and federal health officials, contributed to a healthier South.

After the epidemic, it became clear that Mississippi was, like other southern states, teetering on a seesaw of decision making. Advocates of states' rights believed that only those locals familiar with the peculiar problems of the South should administer health care and distribute relief aid. On the other hand, some southerners believed that local officials were too invested economically in the region and would therefore be unable to administer quarantines properly. Regardless of the political choice, the most important legacy of the 1878 yellow fever epidemic for Mississippi was the mind-set—created through controversy and compromise—that the state needed federal assistance to address overwhelming medical problems. With that understanding, local organizations and a populace with a memory of devastating epidemics could incorporate assistance programs into Mississippi's health care agenda. The implementation of better public health standards in Mississippi would not be easy, as indicated in the early twentieth century when hookworm disease and pellagra were addressed by the U.S. Public Health Service and Rockefeller Foundation monies.[30] Yet one result of the 1878 yellow fever epidemic was an emerging public health care program—one that would grow and come into its own in the twentieth century. As John Ellis noted, "the southern yellow fever epidemic of 1878 stands as . . . a major historical landmark in the development of public health in both region and nation."[31] The story of Mississippi during this pivotal epidemic is a tale of destruction, incompetence, and failing, as well as one of compassion, charity, and reaffirmation of values. And it provided a fertile field for the creation of an effective system of public health that would make such catastrophes rare in the future.

Notes

Preface

1. *Vicksburg Weekly Herald,* October 18, 1878.

2. Ibid., October 17, 1878.

3. Underwood and Whitfield, *Brief History of Public Health,* 1–8.

4. Lowery and McCardle, *History of Mississippi,* 20–25; Fant and Fant, *History of Mississippi,* 38; Sullivan and Powell, *Mississippi Gulf Coast,* 15; Howell, "The French Period," 118–19; Claiborne, *Mississippi as a Province,* 27. In 1706, Iberville himself died of yellow fever in Havana, Cuba.

5. J. M. Keating, *History of the Yellow Fever,* 77–98. Keating outlines the New World's record of yellow fever visitations and refers to the disease by its various names. He also states that in 1596 the first colonial record of yellow fever appears in Central America. By 1618 the disease appeared along the Atlantic Coast and continued unchecked in various North American cities until his report in 1879. Keating states that in 1699, as the French colonized the Mississippi region, Philadelphia experienced a yellow fever epidemic that resulted in two hundred deaths. He records that in 1802, Biloxi, Mississippi, was the site of the first appearance of the disease along the Gulf Coast in the United States.

6. "President's Report," in *Report of the Mississippi State Board of Health,* n.p.

7. See Carrigan, *The Saffron Scourge,* 76–80, for an overview of the creation of and quarantine powers of the Louisiana State Board of Health.

8. Dromgoole, *Dr. Dromgoole's Yellow Fever,* 106.

9. Rosenberg, *Explaining Epidemics,* 281. Rosenberg outlines the definition of an epidemic and the subsequent medical and public response from a historical perspective. He likens past epidemics of all types to the 1980s AIDS scare as a basis for understanding the "patterns of social response."

10. For information regarding other states' experiences and responses to the 1878

yellow fever epidemic, see Bloom, *Great Yellow Fever Epidemic;* and Carrigan, *The Saffron Scourge.*

11. The historical literature on Reconstruction is vast. The traditional view is found in Dunning, *Reconstruction,* and Bowers, *The Tragic Era.* In the 1930s, W. E. B. DuBois challenged the traditional interpretation in *Black Reconstruction.* By the 1960s, revisionist works such as Stampp, *The Era of Reconstruction,* and Franklin, *Reconstruction after the Civil War,* offered new interpretations. More recent comprehensive works include Foner's *Reconstruction: America's Unfinished Revolution.* Cresswell's *Multiparty Politics in Mississippi* explores the growth of third parties such as the Greenbacks and Populists in the political atmosphere of post-Reconstruction Mississippi, and Hyman's *The Anti-Redeemers* outlines sociopolitical class struggles in the aftermath of Reconstruction. McMillen's *Dark Journey* outlines African-American experiences in the state from Reconstruction through the Jim Crow years. Harris provides a comprehensive overview of Reconstruction in Mississippi in *The Day of the Carpetbagger.*

12. McMillen, *Dark Journey,* 38–39.

13. See Harris, "Formulation of the First Mississippi Plan"; Foner and Mahoney, *America's Reconstruction,* 75.

14. *Jackson Clarion,* January 18, February 12, 1868.

15. Garner, *Reconstruction in Mississippi,* 341; Bond, *Political Culture,* 165–68; Craven, *Reconstruction,* 274–84. Craven provides a national view of the 1868 election.

16. Grenada Relief Committee to Governor John M. Stone, August 22, 1878, John Marshall Stone Papers, Mississippi Department of Archives and History, Jackson.

Chapter 1

1. Harris, *Presidential Reconstruction,* 26–27; Wharton, *The Negro in Mississippi,* 13; Bond, *Political Culture,* chapter 4, "The Distressing Influence of War," 118–50.

2. Wharton, *The Negro in Mississippi,* 69–73; McMillen, *Dark Journey,* 123–50. Regarding the "New Servitude" created after the Civil War, McMillen writes: "Black Mississippians also understood the force of tradition. Whatever their expectations at the moment of emancipation, all but a relative few remained subject to the will of the white landlords. Except for the estimable technicality of citizenship, the patterns of their lives were little changed" (124). Even though he primarily examines the black experience in the twentieth century, McMillen traces the history of sharecropping and the crop-lien system from emancipation.

3. Wharton, *The Negro in Mississippi,* 70–73; Harris, *Presidential Reconstruction,* 173.

4. Harris, *Presidential Reconstruction,* 167–72. Harris explains that northern-

ers who remained in or came to Mississippi during and after the Civil War participated in cotton growing and in business opportunities, including professions. After
the Civil War, "The greatest amount of money came to Mississippi with Federal soldiers and Northern immigrants" (169).

5. Wharton, *The Negro in Mississippi*, 164–66; Camejo, *Racism, Revolution, Reaction*, 84–88.

6. The three men arrested were J. Aaron Moore, William Clopton Dennis, and
Warren Tyler.

7. Wharton, *The Negro in Mississippi*, 188–90; Garner, *Reconstruction in Mississippi*, 349–51. In Wharton's account, Sturgis's store burned.

8. Loewen and Sallis, *Mississippi Conflict and Change*, 156.

9. *Slave Narratives*, 104.

10. Wharton, *The Negro in Mississippi*, 190.

11. Garner, *Reconstruction in Mississippi*, 372–95.

12. Ibid., 391–95.

13. See Lowery and McCardle, *A History of Mississippi*, 406–12, for a listing of
the Impeachment Articles as explained in 1890 Mississippi; Bond, *Political Culture*,
181–82.

14. Coker, *Valley of Springs*, 36–37. Stone served another six-year term as governor from 1890 to 1896 and was the president of Mississippi State University (Agricultural and Mechanical College) from 1896 until his death, in 1900.

15. Stone volunteered in the "Iuka Guards," Company K, Second Mississippi
Volunteer Regiment. That regiment later became part of General Joseph R. Davis's
Brigade in the Army of Northern Virginia.

16. Riggs, "Administration of Governor John Marshall Stone," 33–38; Sansing,
"Congressional Reconstruction," 588–89; White, "Mississippi Confederate Veterans,"
147–55; *Jackson Weekly Clarion*, December 5, 1877; Revels, "Redeemers, Rednecks
and Racial Integrity," 595–96; Sumners, *Governors of Mississippi*, 40–50.

Chapter 2

1. Wiltshire, *Mississippi Newspaper Abstracts*, 2:72; Berkow, *Merck Manual*, 57,
764; Carrigan, *The Saffron Scourge*, 4.

2. Warren, "Landmarks in the Conquest of Yellow Fever," 5; Augustin, *History of Yellow Fever*, 85–130, 649; Carter, *Yellow Fever*, 81–197; Bloom, *Great Yellow
Fever Epidemic*, 2–3; J. M. Keating, *History of the Yellow Fever*, 14; Parkes, *A History
of Mexico*, 15. Augustin asserts that Mexico, Central America, and the Caribbean Is-
lands were "the original cradle of the awesome scourge." Parkes also suggests the
possibility that in the ninth century a plague of yellow fever or malaria could have
caused the abrupt cessation of Mayan art and architecture. Carter, on the other hand,

argues that yellow fever originated in West Africa and crossed the Atlantic aboard slave ships throughout the early 1600s. There is also some controversy about the date of yellow fever's appearance in Cuba. Keating states it was in 1620, while Carter believes it was in 1648.

3. Carter, *Yellow Fever,* 4–5; McNeill, *Plagues and Peoples,* 213; Dr. Donald Norris, "Ecology of Vector-Borne Diseases in Man," lecture notes from Parasitology Class at the University of Southern Mississippi, Hattiesburg, 1975.

4. Carter, *Yellow Fever,* 4; Berkow, *Merck Manual,* 54–58; Carrigan, *The Saffron Scourge,* 284. Thirty-eight species of mosquitoes have been infected with the yellow fever virus, but *A. aegypti* is the principal vector. See Belding, *Textbook of Clinical Parasitology,* 808.

5. Holliday, "Remarks of Dr. D. C. Holliday," 207. Holliday recorded these temperatures at the Charity Hospital in New Orleans during the 1878 epidemic. He indicated that both patients were in "profound" comas and died within two hours. Also, the 1878 technological instruments to measure temperatures accurately probably affected these readings.

6. Gazzo, *Yellow Fever Facts,* 6.

7. Stone, *History of the Mild Yellow Fever,* 553.

8. Summers, *Yellow Fever,* 47.

9. Carrigan, *The Saffron Scourge,* 8; Hardenstein, *Epidemic of 1878,* 30; Dromgoole, *Dr. Dromgoole's Yellow Fever,* 39.

10. Daniel, "Original Communications," 2–4.

11. Ibid.

12. Berkow, *Merck Manual,* 57–58; Hardenstein, *Epidemic of 1878,* 86.

13. Hardenstein, *Epidemic of 1878,* 45.

14. Quinine is a white, slightly crystalline bitter alkaloid contained in cinchona barks. It is largely used in medicine because of its tonic and fever-fighting qualities, especially in malaria. Spanish priests during the seventeenth century discovered its curative powers while living in the Andes of Peru. Cinchona bark is harvested from any of various Peruvian trees and shrubs (genus *Cinchona*). The bark yields quinine and related alkaloids. Overdoses of quinine could result in cinchonism, an abnormal condition characterized by giddiness, buzzing in the head, deafness, and temporary loss of sight. See Dobelis, *Magic and Medicine of Plants,* 385–86.

15. Notebook of Dr. Gibson, n.d., 98–99, 285, possession of Mr. Jackie Burkhalter, Glen Allen, Mississippi; Dobelis, *Magic and Medicine of Plants,* 251.

16. T. Cook, *Samuel Hahnemann,* 40; Kaufman, *Homeopathy in America,* 23–47; Dobelis, *Magic and Medicine of Plants,* 65. The first homeopathic college in the United States was the Allentown Academy, established in 1835 by Constantine Hering, a German physician practicing homeopathy in Pennsylvania.

17. *Medical and Surgical Directory,* 3–5.

18. Hardenstein, *Epidemic of 1878,* 92; *North American Homeopathic Directory,* 54. The directory lists Drs. B. D. Chase and F. A. W. Davis, who practiced in Natchez (Adams County), and Drs. Cook, T. J. Harper, A. O. H. Hardenstein, Earnest Hardenstein, Tilford Pegram, John Haszinger, H. R. Pease, and Martin Gilmon, who practiced in Vicksburg (Warren County). Additionally, Dr. C. S. Woodmouse was in Aberdeen (Monroe County), Dr. J. B. Smith was in Camden (Madison County), Dr. James S. Douglas was in McComb (Pike County), Dr. W. J. Gibson was in Fayette (Jefferson County), Dr. William Tegarden was in Mississippi City (Harrison County), and Dr. A. J. Coleman was in Rodney (Jefferson County).

19. Hardenstein, *Epidemic of 1878,* 37.

20. Ibid., 87, 96, 105.

21. Ibid., 92.

22. Ibid., 45.

23. Thomson, *New Guide to Health,* 10–11.

24. Berman and Flannery, *America's Botanico-Medical Movements,* 69–70.

25. First quoted in ibid., 75.

26. Ibid., 70.

27. Haller, *Medical Protestants,* 162–63.

28. J. M. Keating, *History of the Yellow Fever,* 70.

29. F. Peyre Porcher, "Letter to Journal," *Louisville Medical News,* September 28, 1878, 163.

30. R. W. Mitchell, "The Treatment of Yellow Fever," *Louisville Medical News,* November 2, 1878, 215.

31. Hardenstein, *Epidemic of 1878,* 93–94.

32. Livingston, *Cause of and Remedy for Yellow Fever,* 1–2, 9–10. Livingston based his recommendation of the hartshorn plant, a perennial native to North America, upon traditional medicinal botanical knowledge. Native Americans used the hartshorn plant or pasque-flower's sepals to stop nosebleeds, while the leaves relieved rheumatism.

33. *Cincinnati Lancet and Clinic* 1 (1878): 225–30.

34. Duffy, *From Humors to Medical Science,* 85.

35. Quoted in Berman and Flannery, *America's Botanico-Medical Movements,* 25; see Haller, *Medical Protestants,* 31–65, for a detailed explanation of the Thomsonian appeal.

36. Monette, *Observations on the Epidemic Yellow Fever,* 62. The miasmic theory was the leading explanation of yellow fever transmission in the 1853 epidemic as well as the rationale for all fevers. "Bad air" was a catchall phrase to explain the unknown.

37. *In Memoriam: James Busby Norris, M.D.,* 10, 13. Dr. Norris volunteered for medical duty in Vicksburg during the epidemic. He worked for the Howard Association in that city. He was from Chattanooga, and when he died on September 9, 1878, the Masons published this compilation of his correspondence from Vicksburg during his time caring for the city's yellow fever victims and letters of tribute extolling his selfless act of volunteerism. Vicksburg officials buried him in that city, but Secretary of War George N. McCrary later asked that Norris's body be interred in the Chattanooga National Cemetery. Because of the unusual circumstances in the epidemic, military officials gave special consideration to his interment in the national cemetery.

38. In fact, the *Conclusions of the Board of Experts* maintained that fomites carried yellow fever. This board met in Washington, D.C., in January 1879. Members were Isham G. Harris, chairman of the Senate committee; Stanley Matthews of the Senate subcommittee; Casey Young, chairman of the House committee; Dr. John M. Woodworth, surgeon general; and Dr. Chaille of New Orleans, secretary of the committee. Woodworth chaired the Board of Experts, which concluded that "yellow fever should be dealt with as an enemy which imperils life and cripples commerce and industry" and asked for the creation of a central authority "to gain strength from, and give strength to, State and municipal health organizations" (2–3).

39. Dromgoole, *Dr. Dromgoole's Yellow Fever,* 7: Carrigan, *The Saffron Scourge,* 262; Kilpatrick, "An Account of the Yellow Fever," 42.

40. Dromgoole, *Dr. Dromgoole's Yellow Fever,* 11, 44; Zinn, *A People's History,* 259–61. Dromgoole compiled several doctors' opinions regarding the cause and treatment of yellow fever.

41. See Horsman, *Josiah Nott of Mobile,* 150–69. Nott had suggested the mosquito as a vector for yellow fever. He lost four of his children to the disease in the 1853 Mobile epidemic and is buried along with six of his children in Mobile's Magnolia Cemetery. Approximately fifteen hundred years ago, Sanskrit literature suggested mosquitoes as carriers of malaria. See G. Williams, *The Plague Killers,* 107. For information on Texas fever (cattle tick fever) see Ristic and Kreier, *Babesiosis,* and Haley, "Texas Fever and the Winchester Quarantine."

42. *Jackson Daily Bulletin,* September 27, 1897, in Yellow Fever Subject File (1897–1989), Mississippi Department of Archives and History, Jackson.

Chapter 3

1. See Duffy, *Sword of Pestilence,* 44–145. Even though Duffy's work details the New Orleans epidemic, it provides information germane to the overall understanding of epidemic stages.

2. Hildreth, "Early Red Cross," 61; Sullivan and Powell, *Mississippi Gulf Coast,* 61; DeBow, *Statistical View of the United States,* 342 and 371. In 1850 New Orleans's population was 116,375 and Biloxi's was 1,700; see Duffy, *Sword of Pestilence.*

3. Gillson, "Louisiana State Board of Health," 60–61.

4. Susan Alexander Simpson Kate Simpson, August 20, 1878, Kate Simpson Papers, Southern Historical Collection, University of North Carolina, Chapel Hill.

5. Josiah C. Trent, "Eighteenth-Century Physicians and the Yellow Fever," in Smith, *Yellow Fever in Galveston,* 91–92. Trent provides an overview of eighteenth-century physicians who made "small gains" in the understanding of yellow fever. See also Powell, *Bring Out Your Dead,* which provides an account of Philadelphia's 1793 yellow fever outbreak while outlining efforts of contemporary physicians, especially Benjamin Rush.

6. Smith, *Yellow Fever in Galveston,* 16.

7. Cross and Wales, *Atlas of Mississippi,* 44–45.

8. Ibid. Vicksburg's population increased from 3,158 in 1860, to 12,443 in 1870, to 11,814 in 1880, and to 13,373 in 1890, while Meridian grew from a small settlement in 1860, to 2,709 in 1870, to 4,008 in 1880, and to 10,624 by 1890. These figures include both whites and African Americans. *Tenth Census of the United States,* 421.

9. Bond, *Political Culture,* 202–3; Cross and Wales, *Atlas of Mississippi,* 44. See chapter 6 in Bond's book for a complete outline of Mississippi's railroad expansion after the Civil War.

10. C. L. Henderson [?] to J. B. Crowder, October 20, 1878, in possession of author. The signature on the letter is blurred, making the author's name questionable, but the remainder of the letter is clear. It is likely that the author was returning home to Louisville. However, the exact Louisville is unknown, and additional research did not reveal the answer.

11. *Jackson Daily Clarion,* March 6, 1878, in Yellow Fever Subject File (1878), Mississippi Department of Archives and History, Jackson.

12. Ellis, *Yellow Fever and Public Health,* 38–39; Bloom, *Great Yellow Fever Epidemic,* 88; Carrigan, *The Saffron Scourge,* 114; Thomas, *Cuba,* 242–70. Ellis, Bloom, and Carrigan agree that logically the importation of the yellow fever virus in 1878 could have come from any number of sources of contagion. Dr. Choppin vacillated about the role of the *Emily B. Souder* in the 1878 New Orleans yellow fever epidemic. At one point he emphatically stated in a message to the surgeon general of the U.S. Marine Hospital Service, "We are endeavoring diligently to trace the origin of this outbreak, but so far find no connection with any foreign source. *It is clear that they have not resulted from the two cases which were developed two months ago on the steamer Emily B. Souder.*" He composed this message in July and had it published in the *New Orleans Daily Picayune* on July 26, 1878. Later, however, Choppin blamed

the chain of cases from the *Souder*. Carrigan discusses this in *The Saffron Scourge,* 114–15.

13. Ellis, *Yellow Fever and Public Health,* 39; Humphreys, *Yellow Fever and the South,* 28; Bloom, *Great Yellow Fever Epidemic,* 86–87; Carrigan, *The Saffron Scourge,* 114, 78; *New Orleans Daily Picayune,* July 25, 1878; Hardenstein, *Epidemic of 1878,* 1–5.

14. Ellis, *Yellow Fever and Public Health,* 39.

15. Hardenstein, *Epidemic of 1878,* 1–4.

16. Ellis, *Yellow Fever and Public Health,* 39–40; Jones, "Yellow Fever Epidemic of 1878," 605–7; *New Orleans Daily Picayune,* July 24, 28, and 30, 1878.

17. *Laws of the State of Mississippi, 1878,* 129.

18. Bond, *Political Culture,* 225–26.

19. See *Conclusions of the Board of Experts,* 15–16; Bond, *Political Culture,* 225–32.

20. *Laws of the State of Mississippi, 1878,* 134–36.

21. *Report of the Mississippi State Board of Health,* 18–19.

22. *Laws of the State of Mississippi, 1878,* 137. Sec. 19 of an act to amend an act titled "an Act to create a State Board of Health for the Protection of life and health and to prevent the spread of disease in the State of Mississippi, and other purposes," states, "That all incorporated towns in the State shall have the power to pass sanitary laws and to create boards of health, and to suppress as nuisances anything that is dangerous to the public health, with full powers of enforcing ordinances for registration and mortuary statistics."

23. *New Orleans Daily Picayune,* September 10, 1878.

24. *Report of the Mississippi State Board of Health,* 19–20; *New Orleans Daily Picayune,* July 29 and 30, 1878. On July 31, 1878, Johnston sent letters to the mayors of McComb City, Brookhaven, Bogue Chitto, Beauregard, Grand Gulf, Crystal Springs, and Hazlehurst.

25. *Laws of the State of Mississippi, 1878,* 129–37.

26. J. M. Keating, *History of the Yellow Fever,* 95.

27. Ibid.

28. Hardenstein, *Epidemic of 1878,* 27; Records of Frank J. Fisher Funeral Home, 1875–1878, Old Vicksburg Courthouse and Museum, Vicksburg, Mississippi. Stoltz's entry reads as follows: "Paul Stoltz, 26 years, 1 mo. 9 days, Yellow Fever, Sick in Hill City Infirmary, Coffin Box grave Drayage Box use of, Hearse & Servises [*sic*] $45.00, Burial Robe $10.00" (384). The total cost of Stoltz's funeral was $55. Someone paid $44 cash but failed to make the final payment of $11. According to the records, the outstanding balance for his funeral remains unpaid.

29. William H. Hardy to Hattie Lott Hardy, July 31, 1878, Hardy Papers, McCain Library and Archives, University of Southern Mississippi, Hattiesburg.

30. *Pascagoula Democrat-Star,* July 26, 1878.

31. Ibid.

32. The waters at Cooper's Well were believed to cure malaria, dyspepsia, kidney ailments, and skin diseases. As one contemporary physician noted, after drinking the water, "the effects upon the brain are very similar to those that follow the drinking of a few glasses of champagne wine." Personal papers of Colonel and Mrs. Frank Cannon, Long Beach, Mississippi. Mrs. Cannon's family, the Spenglers, purchased Cooper's Well in 1884. She and her husband provided much information about the resort. The Spenglers lost three sons to yellow fever during the 1878 epidemic. The family lived in Vicksburg during that time prior to moving to Raymond and Cooper's Well. The sons who died were William Albert (August 30), Joseph A. (September 18), and Charles Alexander (October 8, 1878); they are buried in the Vicksburg City Cemetery.

33. Interview with and personal papers of Mrs. Genevieve Wilde Barksdale, Ocean Springs, Mississippi. Mrs. Barksdale's collection of family papers includes a letter written by John L. Dennis about his experiences with the shotgun quarantine officers. Cooper's Well was located near present-day Raymond. Mr. and Mrs. B. W. Griffith were ultimately married on May 7, 1879, and celebrated their fiftieth wedding anniversary in Jackson on May 7, 1929. Dennis saw the anniversary announcement in the local Jackson paper and recorded his reminiscence about the quarantine letter. He then sent the letter to the Griffiths as a present. That letter remained in the family as a memento of the occasion.

34. Barksdale interview, September 17, 1995.

35. Ibid.

36. *New Orleans Daily Picayune,* September 7, 1878; *Pascagoula Democrat-Star,* September 20, 1878.

37. *Report of the Mississippi State Board of Health,* 76.

38. *Pascagoula Democrat-Star,* August 30, September 6, 13, 20, and 27, and October 4, 1878; *Baptist Record,* October 31, 1878; Cabaniss, *The University of Mississippi,* 85; Minutes of the Board of Trustees, 1860–1882, University of Mississippi Archives, Special Collections, Oxford.

39. *Pascagoula Democrat-Star,* August 30, 1878.

40. *Report of the Mississippi State Board of Health,* 66–67.

41. Headley, *Claiborne County, Mississippi,* 152–54; *Pascagoula Democrat-Star,* September 6, 1878; *Report of the Mississippi State Board of Health,* 66–67.

42. *Pascagoula Democrat-Star,* September 6, 1878.

43. Ibid., August 2, 1878.

44. Ibid.

45. Albert Buford to Mary Buford, August 8 and 10, 1878, Buford Letters, private collection of Wally Norway, Jackson, Mississippi. The daily correspondence of Albert G. and Mary Buford exemplifies the effects of the yellow fever epidemic in a very emotional manner. Their letters began upon Mary's arrival on the coast on

August 2 and ended with her death on September 9. The Bufords' letters reveal a wealth of information about the cities of Ocean Springs and Water Valley. More importantly, they outline the effects of the epidemic and quarantines in these areas in a personal manner. This couple demonstrated a devotion to each other and a loving concern for one another's health.

46. Albert Buford to Mary Buford, August 8, and Mary Buford to Albert Buford, August 16, 1878, ibid.

47. Mary Buford to Albert Buford, August 21, 23, and 25, 1878, ibid.

48. Mary Buford to Albert Buford, August 29, September 5, 1878, ibid.

49. Telegram, private collection of Wally Norway, Jackson, Mississippi.

50. *Conclusions of the Board of Experts,* Provisional Table 2.

51. Works Progress Administration Historical Project, "Source Material for Mississippi Health History: Hancock County," 1937, Binder 17, M. James Stevens Collection, Biloxi Public Library; Roberts, *Lake Pontchartrain,* 168; *New Orleans Daily Picayune,* July 27, 1878; Dromgoole, *Dr. Dromgoole's Yellow Fever,* 107.

52. *Pascagoula Democrat-Star,* August 2, 1878. Present at the health board meeting in late July were E. F. Griffin, H. L. Howze, S. A. McInnis, D. M. Dunlap, S. R. Thompson, and M. M. Evans. These were businessmen and professionals in Scranton and therefore of the social elite.

53. Lowery and McCardle, *History of Mississippi,* 407–9.

54. *Pascagoula Democrat-Star,* August 2, 1878.

55. Ibid., August 2 and 9, 1878.

56. "Quarantine Station on Ship Island, Mississippi," 1971, Binder 17, Stevens Collection.

57. *New Orleans Daily Picayune,* August 4, 1878; *Pascagoula Democrat-Star,* August 2, 1878. The *Daily Picayune* contained "Coastwide Correspondence" as a travel-interest article for the paper. The authors simply called themselves "Two Boy Passengers." This article provides insight into the quarantine problems faced by ships traveling to the Mississippi Gulf Coast during the 1878 epidemic. The Jackson County Board of Health publicly endorsed Dr. Blount's actions in a meeting on August 5 and printed that endorsement in the August 9 *Pascagoula Democrat-Star.*

58. *Pascagoula Democrat-Star,* August 2 and 9, 1878.

59. Ibid., August 2, 1878.

60. Ibid.

61. Ibid., August 2 and 9, 1878; Sullivan and Powell, *Mississippi Gulf Coast,* 41–69. Sullivan and Powell explore the benefits shared between New Orleans and the Mississippi Gulf Coast, including the influence of yellow fever on the relationship between these two regions.

62. *Pascagoula Democrat-Star,* August 23, 1878.

63. Ibid., August 16, 1878.

64. Bond, *Political Culture,* 110, 197. Bond states that the Mississippi Central, a line between Jackson and the Tennessee border, "lost equipment valued at $750,000." Repairing and replacing this equipment apparently was slow immediately after the Civil War but was accomplished by the time of the 1878 epidemic.

65. *Catholic Advocate* 10 (1875): 23–24, in Yellow Fever Miscellaneous Collection, Marshall County Museum, Holly Springs, Mississippi. This collection includes copies of newspaper and journal articles, letters, and photocopied material on a variety of topics relevant to Marshall County and Holly Springs.

66. Federal Writers' Project of the Works Progress Administration, *Mississippi,* 203.

67. *New York Herald,* September 4, 1878. The *Herald* also reported that "Two companies stationed at Little Rock, Ark., have also been ordered to a place called Dardanelles, about twenty miles distant."

68. Dromgoole, *Dr. Dromgoole's Yellow Fever,* 115; *New Orleans Times,* August 13, 1878.

69. Dromgoole, *Dr. Dromgoole's Yellow Fever,* 115; Power, *The Epidemic of 1878,* 168; J. M. Keating, *History of the Yellow Fever,* 244; McCroskey to Moore, August 26, 1878, Yellow Fever Miscellaneous Collection, Marshall County Museum, Holly Springs, Mississippi. McCroskey wrote this letter to his friend Dr. John R. Moore, who lived north of Holly Springs and was perhaps not in the range of published town news. Some discrepancy exists about the initials of the first man who died in Holly Springs. Dromgoole states that L. L. Downs was the man's name, while Keating and Power state that E. L. Downs was the first fatality. All three agree, however, that Downs was a refugee from Grenada. Also listed in the death rolls of Keating's book is an H. A. McCroskey, who died on September 4, 1878. This man is more than likely the same McCroskey who wrote the letter to Moore.

70. Personal interview with and private papers and artifacts of George Buchanan, Holly Springs, Mississippi, July 20, 1995; personal interview with Minor F. Buchanan, Jackson, Mississippi, July 19, 1995; Dromgoole, *Dr. Dromgoole's Yellow Fever,* 115. George M. Buchanan suffered additional tragedy as a result of the yellow fever epidemic when Victoria Nunnally Buchanan also died of the disease in 1885. After Victoria's death, Buchanan then married Susan Dean, Victoria's cousin. It is from this union that the interviewees trace their ancestry. Both of Buchanan's wives, his three daughters, and two infant sons who were born prior to the 1878 epidemic are buried around the Buchanan monument in Hill Crest Cemetery in Holly Springs.

71. *Yazoo Valley Flag,* November 22, 1878.

72. *New York Herald,* November 7, 1878. See the following pages in Harrison,

Biographical Directory of the American Congress, 1774–1949, for information about the Democrats returned to office: Henry L. Muldrow (1371), James R. Chalmers (677), Otho R. Singleton (1605), Hernando B. Money (1344), and Charles E. Hooker (1072).

73. *Yazoo Valley Flag,* August 13, 1878.

74. Gant, "Yellow Fever in Mississippi," 21–23; *Report of the Mississippi State Board of Health,* 69–72.

75. Gant, "Yellow Fever in Mississippi," 21–23; *Report of the Mississippi State Board of Health,* 70.

76. *Report of the Mississippi State Board of Health,* 69–72.

77. Gant, "Yellow Fever in Mississippi," 21–33.

78. Savitt, "Slave Health and Southern Distinctiveness."

79. C. L. Tilman to Governor Stone, September 14, 1878, John Marshall Stone Papers, Mississippi Department of Archives and History, Jackson.

80. *Jackson Clarion,* September [?], 1878; *Pascagoula Democrat-Star,* September 6 and 27, 1878; *Aberdeen Examiner,* September [?], 1878.

81. *Pascagoula Democrat-Star,* August 30, 1878. The *Democrat-Star* reported statewide cases and deaths throughout the epidemic. The August 30 edition listed the following cities with the case and death numbers at the end of that month: Vicksburg—140 new cases, 25 deaths; Philadelphia—2 cases; Carrollton—1 death. Additionally, J. L. Power frequently listed the dates of cases and deaths in his *The Epidemic of 1878.* The following Mississippi towns were included in his study with deaths occurring by the end of August: Greenville—4; Water Valley—1; Jackson—1; Summit—4 (a father and three of his children); and Osyka—1. Many other Mississippi towns' and villages' deaths are listed in Powers's book, but death numbers are not given for those areas; Powers simply stated that yellow fever was present there. They are as follows: Grenada, Holly Springs, Dry Grove, Lake, Port Gibson, Meridian, Handsboro, Winona, "Valley Home" in Tallahatchie County, Friar's Point, Lebanon, Yazoo City, Cardiff Landing, Bay St. Louis, Senatobia, Horn Lake, Terry, and Cayuga. It is obvious that by the end of August yellow fever could be found in many counties throughout the state and was quickly advancing to epidemic proportions.

Chapter 4

1. C. A. Rice to Gov. John Stone, September 7, 1878, John Marshall Stone Papers, Mississippi Department of Archives and History, Jackson. The members requested a meeting with Stone.

2. Grenada Relief Committee to Gov. J. M. Stone, August 22, 1878, Stone Pa-

pers. The Grenada Relief Committee members were [?] Rish, R. Smith, John Powell, and T. Walton. The four members of the state board of health who met with Governor Stone were C. A. Rice, M. S. Craft, E. Barksdale, and Robert Lowery.

3. Dr. J. D. McRae to Gov. Stone, September 9, 1878, and Stone to McRae, September 10, 1878, Stone Papers.

4. Ellington, *Christ: The Living Water*, 170–72. See Oakes, *Angels of Mercy*, for this order's pivotal role in nursing care.

5. Carrigan, *The Saffron Scourge*, 346–50; Hildreth, "Early Red Cross." The Howards became more or less obsolete after the 1878 epidemic as state boards of health and national agencies expanded their roles in public health. The Howards continued to list themselves as a charitable organization in New Orleans's directories, however, as late as World War I.

6. *Holy Bible*, 13.

7. Power, *The Epidemic of 1878*, 11.

8. *New Orleans Daily Picayune*, August 10, 1847.

9. Ibid., August 12, 1847.

10. Ibid., August 13, 1847.

11. Anderson, "Chapter in the Yellow Fever Epidemic"; Bonner, "The Yellow Plague of '78."

12. Hamilton, "Holly Springs, Mississippi," 83; Ellington, *Christ: The Living Water*, 169–73. Out of the twelve nuns and one Catholic priest who labored in Holly Springs, six of the nuns and Father Oberti died in the epidemic. The six nuns who died were Sisters Stanislaus, Stella, Margaret, Victoria, Lorentia, and Corinthia.

13. See Rosenberg, *The Cholera Years*. Rosenberg explores three epidemics of Asiatic cholera in the United States, concentrating on New York City. He outlines the interaction of medicine and society and how perceptions of disease changed. He also notes the devotion of the Sisters of Charity during the cholera epidemic of 1849. Both the Sisters of Charity and the Sisters of Mercy had a long history of nursing in a variety of epidemics prior to the 1878 yellow fever outbreak.

14. R. M. Swearingen, "Tribute to Sister Corinthia," 1878, Marshall County Museum, Holly Springs, Mississippi; also in Ellington, *Christ: The Living Water*, 172–73.

15. Swearingen, "Tribute to Sister Corinthia." This tribute was in the Marshall County Courthouse until the courthouse underwent renovation in 1926. When the city decided to renovate the building, officials saved the portion of wall with the inscription. Interestingly, at that time the city also returned the wall portion to the Sisters of Charity in Nazareth, Kentucky. When organizers chartered the Marshall County Museum in 1970, the Sisters of Charity loaded the wall piece onto the backseat of a car and drove it to Holly Springs for that city's museum display, thus returning it to its place of origin. It is pertinent to include this tribute in this study in

order to illustrate the depth of devotion to patients and fellow medical workers. They were the heroes of this epidemic.

16. *History of Marshall County, Mississippi;* Ellington, *Christ: The Living Water,* 172–73.

17. *History of Marshall County, Mississippi.*

18. *Holly Springs Occasional,* October 31, 1878. This newspaper reported on that day: "The Relief Committee of Holly Springs has, as if by institution, understood and mastered the situation. Almost overwhelmed by the difficulties, which meet it at every step, in the beginning of the epidemic, it has, reduced every department, for the relief of the sufferers, to a smooth working condition." That day the editors also eulogized Holland, who had died the previous week.

19. See Bond, *Political Culture,* 183–214. Bond discusses the emerging New South economy and its ties to the railroad and retail trade, which were of course linked to racist policies.

20. Anderson, "Chapter in the Yellow Fever Epidemic," 226; H. W. Walter from J. R. Stoutmayd, September 13, 1878, in 1878 Yellow Fever File, Sisters of Charity Archives, Nazareth, Kentucky.

21. Power, *The Epidemic of 1878,* 57.

22. Ibid., 168–69.

23. Governor Z. B. Vance to Stone, September 10, 1878, Stone Papers. On September 17 Stone received a Western Union telegram from William Rockwood, president of the Howard Association in Vicksburg, which stated, "Dr. C. Happoldt has reported here for duty." Power lists Happoldt's death on October 11 at the Yellow Fever Hospital (*The Epidemic of 1878,* 195). His obituary appeared in the *New York Herald* on October 12, 1878.

24. *Cincinnati Commercial,* September 17, 1878.

25. *New York Herald,* September 6, 1878.

26. Ibid., September 1, 1878.

27. Ibid., September 1 and 4, 1878.

28. Holland quoted in Pruitt, *It Happened Here,* 78; and in Power, *The Epidemic of 1878,* 171, 173.

29. McAlexander, *The Prodigal Daughter,* 55–57, 106–19.

30. Ibid., 106–19; Bonner, "The Yellow Plague of '78"; McDowell to Longfellow, September 4, 1878, in Longfellow Collection, Houghton Library, Harvard University, Cambridge, Massachusetts. The Longfellow Collection contains approximately fifty pieces of correspondence that McDowell and Longfellow sent to one another over a period of several years.

31. McAlexander, *The Prodigal Daughter,* 117, 140.

32. Ibid., 116–19; Bonner, "The Yellow Plague of '78"; McDowell to Longfellow, September 4 and 5, 1878, Longfellow Collection.

33. McAlexander, *The Prodigal Daughter,* 116–19; McDowell to Longfellow, September 9, 1878, Longfellow Collection.

34. McDowell to Longfellow, November 28, 1878, Longfellow Collection; Bonner, "The Yellow Plague of '78," 117–18; McAlexander, *The Prodigal Daughter,* 119.

35. Sterling, *Black Foremothers,* 61–66; Wells, *Crusade for Justice,* 9–22. After the 1878 epidemic, Ida Wells moved to Memphis with her remaining six siblings. She cared for them when she was only sixteen years old. She went on to become a dynamic champion of civil rights and anti-lynching legislation. She died on March 25, 1931, leaving behind a legacy of activism.

36. Wells, *Crusade for Justice,* 12.

37. Power, *The Epidemic of 1878,* 169; J. M. Keating, *History of the Yellow Fever,* 245. Keating lists the couple simply as "Jim Wells" and "Mrs. Jim Wells."

38. Anderson, "Chapter in the Yellow Fever Epidemic," 234; Pruitt, *It Happened Here,* 79–84; Power, *The Epidemic of 1878,* 134–36, 169; Legan, "Mississippi and the Yellow Fever Epidemics," 209. On September 17, 1878, Falconer wrote a letter to a friend in Jackson about the situation in Holly Springs: "Oh! The scenes here are beyond human power to describe. I realize that there is One alone who can save. My prayer is made to Him and my Hope is with Him." Quoted in Power, *The Epidemic of 1878,* 134.

39. Power, *The Epidemic of 1878,* 134–36; Harris, "Reconstruction of the Commonwealth"; Sansing, "Congressional Reconstruction," 571–89; Cox, *Dixie's Daughters,* 44–47. Cox distinguishes the New Man of the post–Civil War era but maintains that patrician ideals remained part of the masculine culture of the times.

40. *Starkville Citizen* quoted in Power, *The Epidemic of 1878,* 134–35; (Canton, Miss.) *American Citizen,* September 28, 1878.

41. *Pascagoula Democrat-Star,* November 8, 1878; *New Orleans Daily Picayune,* November 3, 1878; Blum, "Crucible of Disease," 801–3.

42. *Pascagoula Democrat-Star,* September 13, 1878.

43. Dromgoole, *Dr. Dromgoole's Yellow Fever,* 37. See Pillar, "Religious and Cultural Life," 401, for further references to Marshall. Marshall also coordinated relief efforts for the Vicksburg Howard Association.

44. Leavell, *Baptist Annals,* 25.

45. Mayes, "Charles Betts Galloway," 23.

46. King, *The Great South,* 121.

47. Everman and Fort, *History of St. James' Church,* 94–95, 117–23.

48. Ibid., 100, 142–43; King, *The Great South,* 142–43.

49. McMillen, *Dark Journey,* 38–41.

50. Bond, *Political Culture,* 177. Bond discusses this issue in chapter 5, "Political Culture of Racism."

51. L. P. Yerger and Silas McLean to General J. Z. George, Stone Papers.

52. Bond, *Mississippi,* 145.

53. Patrick, *The Reconstruction of the Nation,* 230–33; Simkins, *History of the South,* 326–43.

54. Sabin, *Struggles and Triumphs,* 7.

55. Faust, *Mothers of Invention,* 112.

56. See Sabin, "Unheralded Nurses." Sabin states that men never made up the majority of nurses and that African-American male nurses always had a "subservient role" under the direction of a white male or female if they cared for people outside their own communities. According to statistics she gathered from Dromgoole's *Dr. Dromgoole's Yellow Fever,* 74 males were volunteer nurses during the 1878 yellow fever epidemic, and 20 of those died in the epidemic. An additional 126 male volunteers provided community care as assistants to medical personnel. Sabin writes: "The traditional female domestic role of caring for the sick was transferred to the public male domain when entire communities, commerce, and property were at stake" (58). Certainly, white males had to demonstrate their commitment to the community as providers and as protectors of those who were perceived to be helpless—women, children, and the elderly—while African-American males were freer to volunteer for other reasons besides social expectations.

57. *In Memoriam: James Busby Norris, M.D.,* 7–8.

58. Power, *The Epidemic of 1878,* 192–93. Listed among the Vicksburg dead were four African-American nurses, three of whom accompanied Norris: "Sept. 9, __ Peacock, col.40 y.; Sept. 13, John Johnson, col, 26 y.; Sept. 16, Ed. Massengale, 40 y., Chatanooga [*sic*] nurse." Also, "Sept. 13, Thomas Edwards, col., 36 y. Chattanooga nurse" appeared. Presumably, Edwards joined the group at a later date. No information surfaced on the other nurses. Obviously, record keeping regarding African-American cases/mortality rates was sketchy as the entries do not include Peacock's first name, and officials mistook Massengale's first name, Eldridge, as Ed. (Edward?).

59. *In Memoriam: James B. Norris, M.D.,* 7. The following African-American men volunteered as Howard nurses to accompany Norris: John J. Marshall, Asa Peacock, Eldridge Massingale, John Johnson, Woodson Ellington, Paul Miller, John A. Logan, and Gus Williams. While performing their medical duties in the Vicksburg epidemic, Peacock died on September 9, Norris on September 10, and Johnson on September 13. See Ragland and Renfroe, *Yellow Fever Epidemic of 1878,* 19–41, for a list of all who died in Vicksburg in the 1878 epidemic.

60. Gant, "Yellow Fever in Mississippi," 23. Reed apparently lived through the epidemic, as his name does not appear in Power's or Keating's list of fatalities. See also Sabin, "Unheralded Nurses," 56.

61. *New York Herald,* September 1, 1878.

62. Aunt Minerva Story, loose papers, 1878 Yellow Fever File, Sisters of Charity Archives.

63. Ibid.

64. *Cincinnati Commercial,* September 16, 1878.

65. *Pascagoula Democrat-Star,* November 8, 1878.

66. *New York Herald,* September 4, 1878.

67. Duffy, *Sword of Pestilence,* 344–46.

68. Power, *The Epidemic of 1878,* 182–83.

69. Ordinance quoted in Lord, "Yellow Fever Epidemic of 1878," 27–28.

70. *Report of the Mississippi State Board of Health,* 63–64; Loewen, *The Mississippi Chinese,* 24–25. See also Quan, *Lotus among the Magnolias.* Both Loewen and Quan provide good overviews of the Chinese experience in Mississippi.

71. B. Keating, *History of Washington County,* 55–56.

72. Campbell to Stone, September 21, 1878, Stone Papers.

73. Ibid.; Rousey, "Yellow Fever and Black Policemen," explores another situation where African Americans integrated the white Memphis police force because of the effects of that city's extreme yellow fever experiences.

74. Campbell to Stone, September 24, 1878, Stone Papers.

75. (Canton, Miss.) *American Citizen,* September 28, 1878.

76. *New York Herald,* September 4, 1878.

77. Dillard quoted in Power, *The Epidemic of 1878,* 99.

78. Headley, *Claiborne County, Mississippi,* 153.

79. McMillen, *Dark Journey,* 5.

Chapter 5

1. *Conclusions of the Board of Experts;* Records of Frank J. Fisher Funeral Home, 1875–1878, p. 438, Old Vicksburg Courthouse and Museum, Vicksburg, Mississippi. The Fisher Funeral Home records reflect a citizenry suffering in a horrendous yellow fever epidemic. The people in Vicksburg had to worry about both the disease and dwindling supplies. Because the quarantines had brought business to a standstill, many families could not afford a funeral for their loved ones. The bulk of the entries from pages 404–78 involve yellow fever victims. Because of the dire economic situation in the town, the Howards provided most of these victims a five-dollar funeral.

2. Records of Frank J. Fisher Funeral Home, 1875–1878.

3. Spinzig, *Yellow Fever,* 160; *Conclusions of the Board of Experts,* n.p.; Archer quoted in Power, *The Epidemic of 1878,* 166; Lord, "Yellow Fever Epidemic of 1878," 22; Hemphill, *Fevers, Floods, and Faith,* 105.

4. *Report of the Mississippi State Board of Health,* 53–59; Power, *The Epidemic of 1878,* 177–78; J. M. Keating, *History of the Yellow Fever,* 250.

5. Caire and Caire, *History of Pass Christian,* 27.

6. Personal interview with Nancy K. Williams, Newton, Mississippi, October

19, 1995. Williams was a local historian who had an extensive collection recounting the history of Lake. In that village, the McCallum house still stands just as it did during the 1878 epidemic. It is located across the street from the Methodist church. What is today known as the Kidd house also still exists as it did in 1878. This house is located closest to Lake Cemetery and was the site of several deaths. Captain H. G. McFarland's widow, children, mother-in-law, and sister-in-law all died in the Kidd house. Captain McFarland was one of the six friends who visited Sneed while he recuperated at the Scott house. The other five were Dr. George McCallum, Dr. J. J. Tate, Lee Scott, William H. Evers, and W. E. Crowson. The wives of all of the aforementioned men also died in the epidemic. Lake Cemetery is a grim reminder of the 1878 yellow fever epidemic.

7. Power, *The Epidemic of 1878*, 161–62.

8. Spinzig, *Yellow Fever*, 125–26.

9. Power, *The Epidemic of 1878*, 160–66; Dromgoole, *Dr. Dromgoole's Yellow Fever*, 113–14; *Report of the Mississippi State Board of Health*, 40–46; *Pascagoula Democrat-Star*, September 13, 1878.

10. Coan to Stone, September 18, 1878, telegrams, John Marshall Stone Papers, Mississippi Department of Archives and History, Jackson.

11. Power, *The Epidemic of 1878*, 161–62. The death roll in Grenada reveals a particularly poignant story. Deaths are listed alphabetically, revealing that many people with the same surname died during this epidemic. For example, George W. Lake, Mrs. George W. Lake, Miss Annie Lake, Miss Delia Lake, and Gus Lake are all listed. It is reasonable to conclude that this group is a husband and wife with their children. Modern Grenada records do not tell this story, nor does the contemporary newspaper, the *Grenada Sentinel*. The *Sentinel* did not operate for six weeks during the yellow fever epidemic, but by the end of September it once again began printing. Its first order of business was to list the 214 deaths that had occurred up to that time in the city.

12. Ray, "The Epidemic in Grenada," 45.

13. Carrigan, *The Saffron Scourge*, 255. Carrigan discusses social attitudes concerning race and economic class in chapter 9, pages 234–59. See also Kiple and King, *Another Dimension to the Black Diaspora*, 45–46.

14. Power, *The Epidemic of 1878*, 162; *Report of the Mississippi State Board of Health*, 45.

15. Headley, *Claiborne County, Mississippi*, 153.

16. Personal interview with Edward T. Crisler Jr., September 9, 1995, and private papers of the Crisler family, Port Gibson, Mississippi. Henry Hume Pearson was the sixth child of Charles and Clara Pearson.

17. Dromgoole, *Dr. Dromgoole's Yellow Fever*, 123; *Report of the Mississippi State Board of Health*, 66–69; *Pascagoula Democrat-Star*, September 13 and 27, 1878.

18. Spinzig, *Yellow Fever,* 160; *New York Herald,* September 2, 1878; Power, *The Epidemic of 1878,* 197. The contemporary observer refers to the Civil War and also the military siege of that city that began on May 25, 1863, and ended in surrender on July 4, 1863, when General Ulysses S. Grant was completing the Mississippi Valley campaign and capturing control of the Mississippi River.

19. Power, *The Epidemic of 1878,* 167–68; Lord, "Yellow Fever Epidemic of 1878 in Greenville," 24.

20. *Pascagoula Democrat-Star,* September 27, 1878; *Greenville Times,* September 28, 1878; Power, *The Epidemic of 1878,* 167–68. Ownby, *American Dreams in Mississippi,* 82–109. Ownby explores the development of "New Stores and New Shoppers 1880–1930," illustrating the growth of consumerism in Mississippi in the late nineteenth and early twentieth century. He includes the growth of a woman's market resulting from increased advertisements and innovative store policies.

21. *Greenville Times,* August 24, September 7, 1878; B. Keating, *History of Washington County,* 53–55.

22. B. Keating, *History of Washington County,* 55; *Pascagoula Democrat-Star,* September 6, 1878. The *Greenville Times* on August 24, 1878, reported that the following Greenville citizens were injured in the collapse: "T. W. Warren, leg broken at the ankle; A. C. Patterson, leg broken and both feet dislocated; Henry Levy, thigh broken; Morris Rochelman, one bone of leg broken below the knee; W. E. Hunt and Walter Butler, badly bruised about the back; G. H. Sanford, badly injured; Jonte Equen, badly bruised about the head and back; George Archer, badly bruised about the hip; Charles Moskowitz, Henry Lengsfield, Henry Goldman, I. Moyes, and Grafton Baker, Jr., bruised up; Abe Smith and W. A. Hammer, ankle sprained. Several others suffered slight injuries, and several made narrow escapes. Coming on us at this especial time makes this accident all the more distressing."

23. *Greenville Times,* September 7, 1878.

24. The captain of the steamer *Ben Allen* is quoted in Bloom, *Great Yellow Fever Epidemic,* 129.

25. Power, *The Epidemic of 1878,* 167–68; Spinzig, *Yellow Fever,* 160. Included in the death lists for Greenville in September 1878 are two Chinese men, Sow Lee and Hou Long. By the end of the epidemic, Ways Ah was added to that account. From all indications, these were the only Chinese men who died of yellow fever in Mississippi in 1878. Greenville's mayor was A. B. Trigg; the councilmen were C. E. Morgan, T. P. Perry, and J. H. Sanders; the marshal of the town was John H. Nelson; and Arthur R. Yearger was the attorney. Major Edward P. Byrne was the last official listed on the death rolls.

26. *Pascagoula Democrat-Star,* September 13, 1878.

27. Ibid., September 6 and 13, 1878; Dromgoole, *Dr. Dromgoole's Yellow Fever,* 122.

28. Dromgoole, *Dr. Dromgoole's Yellow Fever,* 117; *New Orleans Daily Picayune,* November 3, 1878.

29. *Pascagoula Democrat-Star,* September 6, 1878.

30. Dromgoole, *Dr. Dromgoole's Yellow Fever,* 114.

31. *Pascagoula Democrat-Star,* September 20, 1878; Power, *The Epidemic of 1878,* 50–51.

32. Power, *The Epidemic of 1878,* 5.

33. Ibid., 19–74. All contributions are listed in this span.

34. Ibid., 19–74; *New York Herald,* September 25, 1878; J. M. Keating, *History of the Yellow Fever,* 248; *Report of the Executive Committee of the Yellow Fever National Relief Commission* lists goods distributed to towns on the Mississippi River; *New York Herald,* September 4, 1878. In *The Epidemic of 1878,* Power meticulously lists every contribution made to Mississippi, charting each town's share of monetary aid and the date it was received.

35. Power, *The Epidemic of 1878,* 28, 42, and 52.

36. *Pascagoula Democrat-Star,* September 6, 1878.

37. Ibid., August 30, September 6, 20, and 27, 1878. Cakes were donated by Mrs. M. A. Dees, Mrs. M. C. Dees, N. Foard, Mrs. Albert Delmas, Mrs. E. Frederick, Misses L. and A. and Mrs. R. P. Blalack, and Mrs. M. Pol. It is interesting to note that these family names are some of the founding ones in the Pascagoula/ Scranton region and that several of them have descendants in the Jackson County area today. Mr. J. Selvas donated cash that was raffled off for the relief cause.

38. Power, *The Epidemic of 1878,* 165–66; Dromgoole, *Dr. Dromgoole's Yellow Fever,* 114. Power quoted Dr. John Brownrigg of Columbus, Mississippi, when he prepared his report about Grenada. Brownrigg described the young telegraph operator in an "oration" before the Mississippi State Medical Association. Unfortunately, Brownrigg failed to mention his name.

39. *Pascagoula Democrat-Star,* October 4, 1878.

40. Blum, "Crucible of Disease," 812, 819–20.

41. Power, *The Epidemic of 1878,* 145. Power lists the following Vicksburg physicians in the death rolls: Drs. Sappington, L. E. Barber, J. B. Norris, Blickfeldt, J. S. Roach, Happoldt, M. C. Blackman, Potts, and Glass (144–46). Two of them in Vicksburg had names spelled two different ways. Blickfeldt also appeared as Blichfeldt, and Happoldt also appeared as Hapholdt. See Ragland and Renfroe, *Yellow Fever Epidemic of 1878,* 19–41, for a list of yellow fever victims in Vicksburg.

42. *Pascagoula Democrat-Star,* September 20, 1878.

43. Headley, *Claiborne County, Mississippi,* 153.

44. *Pascagoula Democrat-Star,* September 27, 1878; E. Merrill to Governor Stone, September 20, 1878, Stone Papers.

45. *Pascagoula Democrat-Star,* September 27, 1878. The *Kosciusko Star* printed

a half sheet during the epidemic, as did the *Magnolia Herald* and the *Corinth Harbinger*. The *Holly Springs Reporter* and the *Holly Springs South* temporarily ceased operation until after the epidemic.

46. Dromgoole, *Dr. Dromgoole's Yellow Fever,* 90.

47. Ibid., 93.

Chapter 6

1. See Carrigan, *The Saffron Scourge,* especially page 284, for an explanation of this cycle as it occurred in Louisiana.

2. Dromgoole, *Dr. Dromgoole's Yellow Fever.* 119; Power, *The Epidemic of 1878,* 179.

3. Dromgoole, *Dr. Dromgoole's Yellow Fever,* 119; Power, *The Epidemic of 1878,* 155, 179.

4. Power, *The Epidemic of 1878,* 154–56.

5. *Pascagoula Democrat-Star,* October 18, 1878; Power, *The Epidemic of 1878,* 155, 179–80; Dromgoole, *Dr. Dromgoole's Yellow Fever,* 120.

6. Spinzig, *Yellow Fever,* 164. The total amount for relief provided to Meridian was $13,631.55. See Power, *The Epidemic of 1878,* 74.

7. Ibid., 163; Ritchie, *Primer of Sanitation,* 160.

8. *Pascagoula Democrat-Star,* October 18, 1878; *Conclusions of the Board of Experts,* appendix; Power, *The Epidemic of 1878,* 187; J. M. Keating, *History of the Yellow Fever,* 246; Dromgoole, *Dr. Dromgoole's Yellow Fever,* 125, 166; Ellington, *Christ: The Living Water,* 492.

9. *Report of the Mississippi State Board of Health,* 82–84.

10. Power, *The Epidemic of 1878,* 183.

11. *Pascagoula Democrat-Star,* October 11 and 25, 1878; *Jackson Clarion,* October 2, 16, and 23, 1878; Spinzig, *Yellow Fever,* 167.

12. Power, *The Epidemic of 1878,* 182–84.

13. For additional information about Jackson in the Civil War see Bearss, *The Battle of Jackson,* 1–135; and Ballard, *Civil War Mississippi,* 62–63, 75.

14. Works Progress Administration Historical Project, "Source Material of Mississippi History: Jackson County," Binder 17, compiled April 4, 1930, Yellow Fever Collection, 1878, M. James Stevens Collection, Biloxi Public Library; *Pascagoula Democrat-Star,* October 4 and 18, 1878. Mullett's grave is in the Krebs Cemetery near Old Spanish Fort in Pascagoula. His epitaph reads: "In Memory of Patrick Mullet, / A resident of Lockport, N. Y. / born in Co. Wexford, Ireland, / March 22, 1843 / Died of yellow fever Oct. 11th, 1878 / Cease weeping dear Mother, Sister, and Brother / I love the place I am sleeping / My time was short, and [bless] the Lord / That called me to his keeping." Even though there are many graves of yellow

fever victims throughout Mississippi, Mullett's epitaph is somewhat unusual in that it names yellow fever as the cause of death.

15. Dromgoole, *Dr. Dromgoole's Yellow Fever,* 122; *Pascagoula Democrat-Star,* October 11, 18, and 25, 1878; Spinzig, *Yellow Fever,* 165.

16. Dromgoole, *Dr. Dromgoole's Yellow Fever,* 122; J. M. Keating, *History of the Yellow Fever,* 249; *Pascagoula Democrat-Star,* October 11, 18, and 25, 1878; Spinzig, *Yellow Fever,* 165.

17. *Pascagoula Democrat-Star,* October 18 and 25, 1878.

18. Dr. Lyon's grave is in the Old Handsboro Cemetery in Gulfport, Mississippi, far from his home.

19. *Pascagoula Democrat-Star,* October 18, 1878.

20. Lawrence, "Three by the Name of Jefferson Davis"; Long, "'My Dear, Manly Son.'"

21. H. Strode, *Jefferson Davis' Private Letters,* 488.

22. Lawrence, "Three by the Name of Jefferson Davis"; Long, "'My Dear, Manly Son'"; H. Strode, *Jefferson Davis' Private Letters,* 487–93; Dromgoole, *Dr. Dromgoole's Yellow Fever,* 84–85.

23. Lawrence, "Three by the Name of Jefferson Davis," 533–35; *Pascagoula Democrat-Star,* October 25, 1878. Another poignant story concerns the death of Jefferson Jr. Apparently, while he was living in Memphis he had asked a "Miss M" to be his wife. He had written to her and stated that he would not "be the football of her caprices" and that she must consent to be his wife or they would no longer see each other. When her reply arrived, he was already stricken with yellow fever and unable to open the letter. Margaret did not read the contents either, and Jefferson Jr. was buried with the unopened letter. "Miss M." later claimed that the letter was an acceptance. Jefferson Jr.'s body was later moved to Hollywood Cemetery near Richmond, Virginia, to be with the rest of the Davis family.

24. The following states recognize an official day for Confederate Memorial Day: Mississippi, Alabama, Georgia, North Carolina, South Carolina, Louisiana, Tennessee (Confederate Decoration Day), Texas (Confederate Heroes Day), and Virginia. For more information on the Lost Cause see Foster, *Ghosts of the Confederacy;* Gallagher and Nolan, *The Myth of the Lost Cause;* and Cox, *Dixie's Daughters.* After the death of Jefferson Davis Jr., his sister Winnie (1864–98) became known as the "Daughter of the Confederacy" and was recognized as the paragon of southern femininity. See C. Cook, "The Challenges of Daughterhood."

25. Quotes in Power, *The Epidemic of 1878,* 136–38; Spinzig, *Yellow Fever,* 181.

26. Power, *The Epidemic of 1878,* 192; Register of Sisters and Loose Paper Collection, Sister Mary Vincent Brown, Private Miscellaneous Collection, 1878, Sisters of Mercy Convent and Archives, Vicksburg, Mississippi; Ellington, *Christ: The Living Water,* 451–52. The Mercy Regional Medical Center in Vicksburg today is the

result of the dedication and hard work of the Sisters of Mercy during the Civil War and the 1878 yellow fever epidemic. The nuns listed on the death rolls in Vicksburg were Mary Regis Grant, Mary Bernadine Murray, Regina Ryan, and Columba McGrath. The convent that was on the hospital's grounds has been moved to Jackson, Mississippi.

27. Cotton, *Asbury: A History,* 29–30. Asbury Cemetery is situated southeast of Vicksburg near the Timberlane Community. Goodrum's statement first appeared in this work.

28. *New York Herald,* October 3, 1878.

29. Hardenstein, *Epidemic of 1878,* 31. Hardenstein records statistics of cases and deaths from pages 26 to 36.

30. *Pascagoula Democrat-Star,* October 18, 1878. Other members of the Handsboro Howards were J. T. Liddle, W. T. Airye, E. B. Myers, General Joseph Davis, and P. K. Mayers.

31. Ibid., October 4, 11, 18, and 25, 1878.

32. Power, *The Epidemic of 1878,* 202–3.

33. *Pascagoula Democrat-Star,* October 11, 1878; "Heroism of the Southern People in War and in Pestilence" quoted from *London Standard* in Power, *The Epidemic of 1878,* 206–7; *Message from the President of the United States to the Two Houses of Congress at the Commencement of the Forty-fifth Congress, with the Reports of the Heads of Departments and Selections from Accompanying Documents* (Washington, D.C.: Government Printing Office, 1878).

34. *Pascagoula Democrat-Star,* October 18, 1878.

35. Dromgoole, *Dr. Dromgoole's Yellow Fever,* 76, 103 (nurse); J. M. Keating, *History of the Yellow Fever,* 248–49.

36. "Miscellany," *Louisville Medical News,* December 7, 1878, 274.

37. *Report of the Executive Committee of the Yellow Fever National Relief Commission.*

38. Ibid., 35–36. The inventory of the *Chambers* included 1,240 shirts, 300 pairs of shoes, 152 tons of ice, 240 undershirts, 1,000 pairs of drawers, 300 pairs of socks, 100 pairs blankets, 5,000 needles, 12 dozen spools of thread, 72 comfort[er]s, 500 pairs of slippers, 48 pounds of Liebig's beef extract, 1,000 bedsacks, 1,000 pillow ticks, 800 dressing gowns, 300 unmade coffins, 372 hats, 350 boxes pilot bread, 300 boxes butter crackers, 5 barrels of rice, 6 coils of rope, 1 barrel of molasses, 12 boxes of corn starch, 10 dozen canned soups, 2 dozen pipes, 10 dozen brooms, 2 dozen clothes brushes, 24 boxes of lemons, 10 cases canned corn, 20 barrels of apples, 60 barrels of potatoes, 10 boxes of candles, 5 dozen scrubbing brushes, 5 kegs of nails, 2 dozen tin dippers, 20 dozen wooden buckets, 6 dozen tumblers, 4 dozen pitchers, 12 dozen yeast powders, 1 case snuff, 2 gross spoons, 16 coops chickens, 600 dozen eggs, 102 barrels of cornmeal, 331 pounds of butter, 33 boxes of cheese, 6 barrels of grits, 1,000

paper bags, 16 boxes of tobacco, 5 pails of tobacco, 60 bags of bacon, 79 barrels of flour, 5 bales of straw, 50 barrels of onions, 1,000 pounds of coffee, 300 pounds of tea, 5 barrels of sugar, 3 cases of matches, 9 sacks of salt, 5 cases of lard, 36 lemon squeezers, 96 pass books [quarantine passage], 24 potato mashers, 27 cases of pepper, 6 barrels of cranberries, 900 pounds of dried beef, 5 cases of clam chowder, 50 cases of mackerel, 10 cases of fish balls, 50 cases of macaroni, 1 barrel of vinegar, 10 boxes of chocolate, 11 cases of mustard, 10 cases of Boston baked beans, 2 cases of cracked wheat, 10 boxes of soap, 20 cans condensed milk, 10 cases of canned peas, 4 half-barrels of pickles, 20 cases of canned tomatoes, 20 cases of corned beef, 2 boxes of clothing, and 1 bale of clothing. This array of provisions suggests that the federal government realized that all aspects of everyday life in Mississippi had been greatly interrupted by the epidemic. No disinfectants were provided, since the epidemic had practically ended in most locations when the *Chambers* embarked for the South.

39. *Pascagoula Democrat-Star,* October 11, 1878; *Report of the Executive Committee of the Yellow Fever National Relief Commission,* 39–41; *Conclusions of the Board of Experts,* n.p.

40. As reported in the *Pascagoula Democrat-Star,* October 11, 1878.

41. *Vicksburg Weekly Herald,* October 11, 1878.

42. Ibid., October 18, 1878.

43. Ibid.

44. J. L. Williams, "Civil War and Reconstruction," 196–202.

45. *Vicksburg Weekly Herald,* October 18, 1878; Ownby, *American Dreams in Mississippi,* 80–81. Ownby shows that black Mississippians by the twentieth century used consumer spending as a means of reshaping their identity from one of subservient worker to one of participant in the American dream of private ownership.

46. Dromgoole, *Dr. Dromgoole's Yellow Fever,* 99. Dromgoole describes a four-story building in the Uptown New Orleans area around Magazine Street from which flour, rice, coffee, tea, sugar, salt, molasses, and salt meat were distributed. Approximately fifteen hundred families received daily provisions from the Peabody Subsistence Association.

47. *Vicksburg Weekly Herald,* October 18, 1878; Carrigan, *The Saffron Scourge,* 120–25. Carrigan provides an overview of benevolent societies and relief efforts in Louisiana in 1878. The Peabody Subsistence Association was charged with racial discrimination during New Orleans's 1878 yellow fever epidemic from the African-American organization called the Mutual Benevolent Relief Association. The Peabody association called the accusations "unfounded" (122–23).

48. *Vicksburg Weekly Herald,* October 18, 1878.

49. Ibid.; loose paper on yellow fever, no author, Miscellaneous Yellow Fever Collection, Old Vicksburg Courthouse and Museum, Vicksburg, Mississippi; *Report of*

the *Executive Committee of the Yellow Fever National Relief Commission,* 34; Blum, "Crucible of Disease," 794.

50. *Vicksburg Weekly Herald,* November 1, 1878.

Chapter 7

1. *Pascagoula Democrat-Star,* November 1 and 8, 1878.

2. R. W. Mitchell, "The Treatment of Yellow Fever," *Louisville Medical News,* November 2, 1878, 214.

3. L. P. Yandell, "The Late Yellow-Fever Outbreak in Louisville," *Louisville Medical News,* December 7, 1878, 277; Uhler, "The Prevention of Yellow Fever," 10–11.

4. Schmidt, "On the Nature of the Poison," 482–83. See also *Cincinnati Lancet and Clinic* 1 (1878): 102; and Woodworth, "Medical News," 160. The contagious aspect of yellow fever had been debated for approximately sixty years. Carrigan discusses this debate in *The Saffron Scourge,* 212–33, 262. Finlay discusses the mosquito as a vector for yellow fever in a paper read before the Royal Academy of Medical, Physical, and Natural Sciences of Havana in 1881: "The Mosquito Hypothetically Considered as an Agent in the Transmission of Yellow Fever." Finlay's theory would not be proved for several years because of the timing factor associated with yellow fever. Carrigan states that "only in the first two or three days of illness is the virus sufficiently concentrated in the patient's blood so that a mosquito can ingest it with a blood meal" (284). The other timing factor involves the ten to fourteen days the virus needs to multiply adequately in the mosquito and travel to her salivary glands, "after which time the mosquito is able to inject the virus while taking another blood meal" (284). As Carrigan states, Finlay was not aware of these timing factors and therefore was initially unsuccessful in laboratory experiments (283–85).

5. Dromgoole, *Dr. Dromgoole's Yellow Fever,* 21–22.

6. G. Williams, *The Plague Killers,* 185–208. Williams traces the conquest of yellow fever. The vaccine for yellow fever, 17D, was successfully developed in 1936. After extensive testing in 1938, the vaccine was mass produced. Dr. Max Theiler, working under the supervision of Dr. Wilber A. Sawyer in the International Health Division of the Rockefeller Foundation, created the vaccine for jungle yellow fever. Urban yellow fever was more controllable through *A. aegypti* habitats. See Shaplen, *Towards the Well-Being of Mankind.*

7. At the Mississippi State Board of Health meeting on November 27, 1879, held to investigate and report on the 1878 yellow fever epidemic and other health matters in the state, many health boards sent representatives to the convocation. Attending were state board of health members, county board of health members, and municipal board of health members. From the Mississippi State Board of Health

were the following: C. A. Rice, president; Wirt Johnston, secretary; F. W. Dancy, at-large member; K. L. Phares, at-large member; Wirt Johnson, at-large member; J. M. Taylor, First District; E. P. Sale, First District; T. D. Isom, Second District; John Wright, Second District; S. V. D. Hill, Third District; B. F. Kittrell, Third District; P. J. McCormick, Fourth District; George E. Redwood, Fourth District; Robert Kells, Fifth District; J. W. Bennett, Fifth District; R. G. Wharton, Sixth District; C. A. Rice, Sixth District. The following county boards of health were represented at the meeting: Alcorn, Attala, Amite, Adams, Benton, Bolivar, Coahoma, Clarke, Choctaw, Covington, Carroll, Claiborne, Clay, DeSoto, Grenada, Hinds, Harrison, Hancock, Holmes, Issaquena, Jefferson, Jasper, Jackson, Kemper, Leflore, Lafayette, Lee, Lowndes, Leake, Lauderdale, Madison, Marshall, Monroe, Marion, Montgomery, Noxubee, Newton, Oktibbeha, Panola, Prentiss, Pontotoc, Rankin, Sharkey, Simpson, Sumner, Tippah, Tate, Winston, Washington, Wilkinson, Yalobusha, and Yazoo. The following municipal boards of health were represented: Austin, Abbeville, Baldwyn, Black Hawk, Byhalia, Batesville, Byram, Beauregard, Benton, Booneville, Cumberland, Cato, Crystal Springs, Coffeeville, Carthage, Concordia, Clinton, Durant, Duck Hill, Enterprise, Holly Springs, Hillsboro, Jackson, Liberty, Lodi, Lake, Louisville, Morton, McComb City, Mt. Pleasant, Magnolia, Macon, Osyka, Okolona, Pleasant Hill, Pickens. Pontotoc, Port Gibson, Rienzi, Rodney, Sardis, Summit, Satartia, Starkville, Taylor's Depot, Vaiden, Verona, Vicksburg, Waynesboro, and Wesson. *Report of the Mississippi State Board of Health,* 1–6.

8. Ibid., 7.

9. Ibid., 7–8.

10. Ibid.

11. Ibid., 5.

12. Ibid., 8.

13. Humphreys, *Yellow Fever and the South,* 64; see pp. 45–76 for a discussion of the National Board of Health and yellow fever.

14. *Mississippi Statistical Summary of Population,* 76; *Tenth Census of the United States,* 421. Included in Vicksburg's 1880 population statistics were 1 Chinese and 2 Indians.

15. *Conclusions of the Board of Experts,* n.p.

16. *Tenth Census of the United States,* 421.

17. Power, *The Epidemic of 1878,* 182; *Conclusions of the Board of Experts,* table 2; Spinzig, *Yellow Fever,* 167; *Mississippi Statistical Summary of Population,* 1. Included in the non-white category were 898 individuals who were not African American.

18. *Conclusions of the Board of Experts,* Provisional Table 2.

19. Power, *The Epidemic of 1878,* 184.

20. Blum, "Crucible of Disease," 801.

21. *Pascagoula Democrat-Star,* November 8, 1878.

22. Wakelyn, *Biographical Dictionary of the Confederacy,* 352; Power, *The Epidemic of 1878,* 101–5. Power's account includes many letters of appreciation from towns and communities throughout Mississippi.

23. Blum, "Crucible of Disease"; Power, *The Epidemic of 1878,* 5–7, 74.

24. Power, *The Epidemic of 1878,* 5–8, 73.

25. Ibid., 100.

26. *Report of the Mississippi State Board of Health,* 5.

27. See McClellan, *McClellan's Own Story,* and Hassler, *General George B. McClellan,* for more information on this former Union general who solicited funds for Mississippi in 1878.

28. R. B. Hubbard, "Proclamation by the Governor," November 12, 1878; George B. McClellan, "Proclamation by the Governor," November 8, 1878; Shelby M. Cullom, "Thanksgiving Proclamation," November 9, 1878; all in John Marshall Stone Papers, Mississippi Department of Archives and History, Jackson.

29. *Report of the Mississippi State Board of Health,* 4–5.

30. *Water Valley Courier,* December 21, 1878; *Holly Springs Reporter,* December 19, 1878; Power, *The Epidemic of 1878,* 112–15.

31. Power, *The Epidemic of 1878,* 115.

32. Ibid., 56–58.

33. *Pascagoula Democrat-Star,* November 8, 1878.

34. Ibid.

35. Ibid.

36. Ibid., November 8, 15, 22, and 29, 1878.

37. *Vicksburg Daily Commercial,* November 15, 1878. Notices in this paper announced the names of returning citizens; e.g., "W. H. Smith and family were among passengers by rail to-day" and "The family of Mr. Laz Hirsh arrived this morning."

Chapter 8

1. Carrigan, *The Saffron Scourge,* 127; Bloom, *Great Yellow Fever Epidemic,* 280.

2. Gant, "Yellow Fever in Mississippi," 23; *Report of the Mississippi State Board of Health,* 2–25. For a list of the physicians who died in the epidemic see Ragland and Renfroe, *Yellow Fever Epidemic of 1878,* 55. Population statistics are from Cross and Wales, *Atlas of Mississippi,* 52.

3. *Crystal Springs Monitor,* December 12, 1878. For further information on public health and the interaction between national and state health boards, see Toner, "Boards of Health in the United States"; Duffy, "Yellow Fever in the Continental United States"; Warner, "Local Control versus National Interest"; and Ellis, *Yellow Fever and Public Health,* 60–82.

4. The committee consisted of Chairman Alexander R. Shepherd, Secretary William Dickson, Treasurer Lewis J. Davis, and members Arthur MacArthur, George Hill Jr., Leonard Whitney, John F. Cook, John W. Woodworth, M.D., John T. Mitchell, A. S. Solomons, Simon Wolf, and B. H. Warner. *Report of the Executive Committee of the Yellow Fever National Relief Commission,* cover page. The committee listed the following cases and deaths in the 1878 epidemic: Louisiana—29,957 cases/5,041 deaths; Mississippi—13,386 cases/3,699 deaths; Tennessee—17,315 cases/ 4,088 deaths; Kentucky—764 cases/366 deaths; Alabama—630 cases/172 deaths; Illinois—100 cases/53 deaths; Ohio—95 cases/40 deaths; Florida—37 cases/17 deaths; Missouri—119 cases/58 deaths. Other sources list different case/mortality numbers. The committee itself stated, "This number probably falls considerably below the actual numbers of cases and deaths" (25–26).

5. Ellis, *Yellow Fever and Public Health,* 61–67.

6. Ibid., 65–66; *New York Times,* November 22, 1878.

7. Ellis, *Yellow Fever and Public Health,* 68.

8. First quoted in ibid., 68–69.

9. Bond, *Political Culture,* 272.

10. See Savitt and Young, *Disease and Distinctiveness,* 29–119. Malaria, yellow fever, hookworm disease, and pellagra all contributed to the notion of an unhealthy South peopled by sickly, lazy citizens.

11. Ellis, *Yellow Fever and Public Health,* 69–75.

12. Ibid., 77–78.

13. Humphreys, *Yellow Fever and the South,* 62–64; Ellis, *Yellow Fever and Public Health,* 75.

14. *Congressional Record,* 46th Cong., 1st sess., vol. 9, pt. 1, p. 72. Woodworth never became the president of the national board, as he died eleven days after its enactment, possibly as a suicide.

15. Humphreys, *Yellow Fever and the South,* 64.

16. *Report of the Mississippi State Board of Health,* 165–79.

17. *Appletons' Annual Cyclopaedia and Register,* 575.

18. Bond, *Political Culture,* 205.

19. *Appletons' Annual Cyclopaedia and Register,* 318.

20. Klein, *History of the Louisville and Nashville Railroad,* 151–52; *New Orleans Daily Picayune,* August 20, November 27, 1878.

21. Hemphill, *Fevers, Floods, and Faith,* 105.

22. Walker, *Tenth Census Report of the Productions of Agriculture,* xviii; McCandless, *Base Book,* 6.

23. McCandless, *Base Book,* 6. See also U.S. Department of Agriculture, *Cotton and Cottonseed,* 14.

24. *Conclusions of the Board of Experts,* 16.

25. Ibid.

26. Hardenstein, *Epidemic of 1878,* 64; *Conclusions of the Board of Experts,* 16.

27. A. T. Semmes, "The Epidemic at Canton, 1878," in *Report of the Mississippi State Board of Health,* 52. See also in that report H. J. Ray, "The Epidemic in Grenada, 1878," 40–46; F. E. Daniel, "Epidemic Yellow Fever at Lake, Miss.," 53–58; F. W. Dancy, "The Epidemic at Holly Springs, Miss., in 1878," 59–63; R. S. Toombs, "The Epidemic at Greenville, 1878," 63–65; R. G. Wharton, "The Epidemic at Port Gibson, 1878," 66–69; H. A. Gant, "The Epidemic at Water Valley, 1878," 69–72; T. H. Gordon, "The Epidemic in Tillatoba and Vicinity, 1878," 79–82; J. M. Calhoun, "The Epidemic at Valley Home, 1878," 85–89; and P. H. Griffin, "Epidemic at Meridian, 1878," 155–59.

28. "A Negro" to Stone, September 26, 1878, John Marshall Stone Papers, Mississippi Department of Archives and History, Jackson.

29. "A Negro" to Stone, January 1879, ibid.

30. See Kraut, *Goldberger's War,* 91–231, for a complete examination of the conquest of pellagra and Mississippi's role in that effort. See Etheridge, *The Butterfly Caste,* 65–217, for an overview of pellagra, its impact on the South, and unlocking the cause of the disease.

31. Ellis, *Yellow Fever and Public Health,* 167.

A Note on Resources

Of all the resources that contribute to the creation of a monograph, primary sources are the infrastructure upon which the work depends. As I worked to complete this project, I was fortunate to have many local and national collections and heretofore untapped primary sources contributed by Mississippians. Without the voices of the citizens who endured the 1878 yellow fever epidemic, the story that unfolds from these multiple resources could never have been told.

Many manuscript collections were vital to this project. The M. James Stevens Collection at the Biloxi Public Library in Biloxi offered good background information about the various epidemics that have affected the Gulf Coast. Local collections such as the Stevens set are found throughout the state and provide good grounding for this regional study. The Marshall County Museum in Holly Springs and the Old Vicksburg Courthouse and Museum were vital in providing intriguing information about the epidemic. Nationally, the Longfellow Collection at Houghton Library at Harvard; the National Library of Medicine at the National Institute of Health in Bethesda; the Sisters of Charity Archives in Nazareth, Kentucky; the Sisters of Mercy Convent and Archives in Vicksburg, Mississippi; and the Edward G. Miner Library, University of Rochester School of Medicine and Dentistry all contained pertinent resources needed to explain yellow fever and its impact on Mississippi. The collection at the McCain Library and Archives at the University of Southern Mississippi contains the William H. Hardy Papers, which provided an interstate perspective. Also, the Miscellaneous Papers about yellow fever at the University of Mississippi Special Collections as well as the Kate Simpson Papers at the Southern Historical Collection at the University of North Carolina, Chapel Hill, all are valuable resources. The Mississippi Department of Archives and History in Jackson possesses a large collection of papers on yellow fever and the John Marshall Stone Papers, which added a good perspective to the study regarding Governor Stone and petitions to him during the epidemic. Each of these collections was instrumental in revealing the hardships and triumphs of Mississippians during the epidemic.

Private collections were as valuable as public resources. Mississippians collect and cherish their family stories, and I was privileged to have several private papers offered for use during my research. Minor F. Buchanan of Jackson shared the George Buchanan Papers, Wally Norway brought to light the Albert G. and Mary Buford Letters (they literally were found in a trunk in an attic), the late Mrs. Genevieve Wilde Barksdale generously allowed me to read Benjamin W. Griffith's diaries, the late Mr. Edward T. Crisler opened his family Bible for me to use, and Colonel and Mrs. Frank Cannon shared the Spengler Family Papers. In addition, Mr. Jackie Burkhalter handed me Dr. Gibson's Prescription Book of 1878 and urged me to use it as I could. The late Nancy K. Williams also shared her knowledge of Lake, Mississippi, and her collection of papers. These Mississippians contributed invaluably to this work through their family histories and knowledge of the state.

Several books of the period were important to this study. J. P. Dromgoole wrote *Dr. Dromgoole's Yellow Fever: Heroes, Honors, and Horrors of 1878,* in which he provides popular remedies, case and death lists, and anecdotal stories about events and personalities in the epidemic. Also, J. M. Keating's *History of the Yellow Fever: The Yellow Fever Epidemic of 1878 in Memphis, Tenn.* cross-referenced monetary contributions and case/death statistics in Mississippi. By far, the most important work explaining the impact of the epidemic on Mississippi is J. L. Power's *The Epidemic of 1878 in Mississippi: Report of the Yellow Fever Relief Work through J. L. Power, Grand Secretary of Masons and Grand Treasurer of Odd Fellows,* which details every aspect of the yellow fever epidemic except medical theories and remedies.

In addition to books, journals of the period were invaluable in adding medical perspective to the study. The *Louisville Medical News, New Orleans Medical Journal,* and *Cincinnati Lancet and Clinic* were the three most significant sources to this study, as were the publications of the Mississippi State Board of Health during and immediately after the epidemic. Moreover, newspapers were often open windows through which local events and reactions to the epidemic could be viewed. The *Jackson Clarion-Ledger* and *Weekly Clarion* as well as the *Vicksburg Weekly Herald* were significant in reporting events throughout Mississippi. The most important newspaper to this study, however, was the *Pascagoula Democrat-Star.* This newspaper is housed in its entirety at the Jackson County Archives. Newspapers from other states that were significant in reporting the epidemic were the *New Orleans Daily Picayune,* the *New Orleans Times,* the *New York Times,* the *New York Herald, Frank Leslie's Illustrated Newspaper,* and the *Memphis Appeal.* Often newspapers outside of the state reported events during the epidemic with a different perspective than the in-state newspapers. Therefore, these papers were important for analysis and comparison.

Both the state of Mississippi and the federal government published vital records of the epidemic that were pertinent to this work. The *Report of the Mississippi State Board of Health for the Years 1878–'79* and two federal reports— *Conclusions of the Board of Experts Authorized by Congress to Investigate the Yellow Fever Epidemic of 1878* and *Report of the Executive Committee of the Yellow Fever National Relief Commission*—were essential in understanding the state and federal recommendations regarding causes, preventatives, and quarantine suggestions after the epidemic.

Secondary sources were central in explaining Mississippi during Reconstruction and afterward. Bradley G. Bond's *Political Culture in the Nineteenth-Century South: Mississippi, 1830–1900,* Eric Foner's *Reconstruction: America's Unfinished Revolution, 1863–1877,* and Neil McMillen's *Dark Journey: Black Mississippians in the Age of Jim Crow* were particularly insightful.

Other secondary sources proved to be fundamental in explaining the medical history of yellow fever epidemics in Mississippi and surrounding states, including Alex Berman and Michael A. Flannery's *American's Botanico-Medical Movements: Vox Populi;* Khaled J. Bloom's *The Mississippi Valley's Great Yellow Fever Epidemic of 1878;* Jo Ann Carrigan's *The Saffron Scourge: A History of Yellow Fever in Louisiana, 1796–1905;* John Duffy's *Sword of Pestilence: The New Orleans Yellow Fever Epidemic of 1853;* John H. Ellis's *Yellow Fever and Public Health in the New South;* and Margaret Humphreys's *Yellow Fever and the South.* Additionally, William H. McNeill's *Plagues and Peoples* offers explanations about the reaction of people to various epidemics on a broad historical scale, and Ronald L. Numbers and Todd L. Savitt's edited volume *Science and Medicine in the Old South* contains articles about antebellum medical history. Charles E. Rosenberg's *Explaining Epidemics and Other Studies in the History of Medicine* also provides explanations of the impact of epidemics, while Todd L. Savitt and James Harvey Young explore yellow fever and other southern diseases in *Disease and Distinctiveness in the American South. Nurses' Work: Issues across Time and Place,* edited by Patricia D'Antonio, includes a good overview about the development of nurses as medical personnel.

Journals also proved to be valuable to this study, The *Journal of Southern History,* the *Journal of Mississippi History,* and *Louisiana History* provided numerous articles including political, economic, and medical explorations related to this study.

These notes do not represent an exhaustive survey of the resources related to yellow fever in Mississippi. However, they do provide a good starting point for researchers who come afterward in exploring this significant event.

Bibliography

Manuscript Collections

Biloxi Public Library, Biloxi, Mississippi
    Stevens, M. James. Collection.
Houghton Library, Harvard University, Cambridge, Massachusetts
    Longfellow Collection.
Marshall County Museum, Holly Springs, Mississippi
    Catholic Advocate, 1875.
    Marshall County and Holly Springs Collection.
    Yellow Fever Miscellaneous Collection.
McCain Library and Archives, University of Southern Mississippi, Hattiesburg
    Agnew, Samuel Andrew. Diary.
    Hardy, William H. and Hattie Lott. Papers.
Edward G. Miner Library, University of Rochester School of Medicine and Dentistry, Rochester, New York
    Miner Yellow Fever Collection.
Mississippi Department of Archives and History, Jackson
    Stone, John Marshall. Papers.
    Yellow Fever Collection, Miscellaneous Papers.
National Institute of Health, National Library of Medicine, History of Medicine Division, Bethesda, Maryland
    Yellow Fever Collection.
Old Vicksburg Courthouse and Museum, Vicksburg, Mississippi
    Miscellaneous Yellow Fever Collection.
    Records of Frank J. Fisher Funeral Home, 1875–1878.
Sisters of Charity Archives, Nazareth, Kentucky
    1878 Yellow Fever File.
Sisters of Mercy Convent and Archives, Vicksburg, Mississippi

Private Miscellaneous Collection, 1878.
Southern Historical Collection, University of North Carolina, Chapel Hill
    Simpson, Kate. Papers.
Special Collections, University of Mississippi, Oxford
    Yellow Fever Miscellaneous Papers—1878.

Newspapers (all 1878 unless noted otherwise)

Mississippi:
Aberdeen Examiner
Baptist Record
Canton American Citizen
Corinth Harbinger
Crystal Springs Monitor
Greenville Times
Holly Springs Occasional
Holly Springs Reporter
Jackson Clarion, 1868
Jackson Clarion-Ledger
Jackson Daily Bulletin
Jackson Weekly Clarion, 1877
Kosciusko Star
Magnolia Herald
Pascagoula Democrat-Star
Starkville Citizen
Vicksburg Daily Commercial
Vicksburg Weekly Herald
Water Valley Courier
Yazoo Valley Flag

Louisiana:
New Orleans Daily Picayune, 1847
New Orleans Times

Ohio:
Cincinnati Commercial

New York:
Frank Leslie's Illustrated Newspaper
New York Herald

Bibliography / 173

New York Times

Tennessee:
Memphis Daily Appeal

Books, Articles, Theses, and Dissertations

Anderson, Mrs. William Albert. "A Chapter in the Yellow Fever Epidemic of
1878." *Publications of the Mississippi Historical Society* 10 (1909): 223–29.
Appletons' Annual Cyclopaedia and Register of Important Events of the Year 1878.
Vol. 3. New York: D. Appleton, 1888.
Augustin, George. *History of Yellow Fever.* New Orleans: Searcy and Pfaff, 1909.
Ballard, Michael B. *Civil War Mississippi: A Guide.* Jackson: University Press of Mississippi, 2000.
Bates, Barbara. *Bargaining for Life: A Social History of Tuberculosis, 1876–1938.*
Philadelphia: University of Pennsylvania Press, 1992.
Bearss, Edwin C. *The Battle of Jackson, May 14, 1863.* Baltimore: Gateway Press,
1981.
Belding, David L. *Textbook of Clinical Parasitology.* New York: Appleton-Century-Crofts, 1952.
Berkow, Robert, ed. *The Merck Manual of Diagnosis and Therapy.* 13th ed. Rahway,
N.J.: Merck, 1977.
Berman, Alex, and Michael A. Flannery. *America's Botanico-Medical Movements:
Vox Populi.* New York: Pharmaceutical Products Press, 2001.
Bettersworth, John K. *Mississippi: A History.* Austin: Steck, 1959.
Bloom, Khaled J. *The Mississippi Valley's Great Yellow Fever Epidemic of 1878.*
Baton Rouge: Louisiana State University Press, 1993.
Blum, Edward J. "The Crucible of Disease: Trauma, Memory, and National Reconciliation during the Yellow Fever Epidemic of 1878." *Journal of Southern History* 69 (November 2003): 791–820.
Boles, John. *Black Southerners, 1619–1869.* Lexington: University Press of Kentucky, 1983.
Bond, Bradley G. *Mississippi: A Documentary History.* Jackson: University Press of
Mississippi, 2003.
———. *Political Culture in the Nineteenth-Century South: Mississippi, 1830–1900.*
Baton Rouge: Louisiana State University Press, 1995.
Bonner, Sherwood. "The Yellow Plague of '78: A Record of Horror and Heroism."
Youth's Companion, April 3, 1879, 117–19.
Bowers, Claude. *The Tragic Era: The Revolution after Lincoln.* Boston: Houghton
Mifflin, 1957.

Cabaniss, Allen. *The University of Mississippi: Its First Hundred Years.* Hattiesburg: University and College Press of Mississippi, 1971.

Caire, R. J., and Katy Caire. *History of Pass Christian.* Pass Christian, Miss.: Lafayette, 1976.

Calhoun, J. M. "The Epidemic at Valley Home, 1878." *Report of the Mississippi State Board of Health for the Years 1878–'79,* 85–89. Jackson, Miss.: Power and Barksdale, 1879.

Camejo, Pedro. *Racism, Revolution, Reaction, 1861–1877: The Rise and Fall of Radical Reconstruction.* New York: Monad Press, 1976.

Carrigan, Jo Ann. *The Saffron Scourge: A History of Yellow Fever in Louisiana, 1796–1905.* Lafayette: University of Southwestern Louisiana Press, 1994.

Carter, Henry Rose. *Yellow Fever: An Epidemiological and Historical Study of Its Place of Origin.* Baltimore: Williams and Wilkins, 1931.

Claiborne, J. F. H. *Mississippi as a Province, Territory and State: With Biographical Notes of Eminent Citizens.* Jackson, Miss.: Power and Barksdale, 1880.

Coker, William L. *Valley of Springs: The Story of Iuka.* Winston-Salem, N.C.: Hunter, 1975.

Conclusions of the Board of Experts Authorized by Congress to Investigate the Yellow Fever Epidemic of 1878, Being in Reply to Questions of the Committees of the Senate and House of Representatives of the Congress of the United States, upon the Subject of Epidemic Diseases. Washington, D.C.: Government Printing Office, 1879.

Cook, Cita. "The Challenges of Daughterhood." In *Mississippi Women: Their Histories, Their Lives,* ed. Martha Swain, Elizabeth Anne Payne, and Marjorie Julian Spruill, 21–38. Athens: University of Georgia Press, 2003.

Cook, Trevor. *Samuel Hahnemann, the Founder of Homeopathic Medicine.* Wellingborough, U.K.: Thorsons, 1981.

Cotton, Gordon. *Asbury: A History; The History of a Church, a Cemetery, and a Community.* Vicksburg, Miss.: privately published, 1994.

Cox, Karen. *Dixie's Daughters: The United Daughters of the Confederacy and the Preservation of Confederate Culture.* Gainesville: University Press of Florida, 2003.

Craven, Avery Odelle. *Reconstruction: The Ending of the Civil War.* New York: Holt, Rinehart and Winston, 1969.

Crawford, John. *A Lecture, Introductory to a Course of Lectures on the Cause, Seat and Cure of Diseases.* Baltimore: Edward J. Coale, 1811.

Cresswell, Stephen. *Multiparty Politics in Mississippi, 1877–1902.* Jackson: University of Mississippi Press, 1995.

Cross, Ralph D., and Robert W. Wales, eds. *Atlas of Mississippi.* Jackson: University Press of Mississippi, 1974.

Dancy, F. W. "The Epidemic at Holly Springs, Miss., in 1878." *Report of the Missis-*

sippi State Board of Health for the Years 1878–'79, 59–63. Jackson, Miss.: Power and Barksdale, 1879.

Daniel, F. E. "Epidemic Yellow Fever at Lake, Miss." *Report of the Mississippi State Board of Health for the Years 1878–'79,* 53–58. Jackson, Miss.: Power and Barksdale, 1879.

———. "Original Communications." *Mississippi Valley Medical Monthly* 2 (1882): 2–4.

D'Antonio, Patricia, et al., eds. *Nurses' Work: Issues across Time and Place.* New York: Springer, 2007.

DeBow, J. D. B. *Statistical View of the United States Embracing Its Territory, Population—White, Free Colored, and Slave—Moral and Social Condition, Industry, Property, and Revenue; The Detailed Statistics of Cities, Towns and Counties; Being A Compendium of the Seventh Census To which Are Added The Results of Every Previous Census, Beginning with 1790, In Comparative Tables, With Explanatory and Illustrative Notes, Based Upon the Schedules And Other Official Sources of Information.* Reprint. New York: Norman Ross, 1990.

Dobelis, Inge N., ed. *Magic and Medicine of Plants.* Pleasantville, N.Y.: Reader's Digest Association, 1993.

Dollard, John. *Caste and Class in a Southern Town.* Madison: University of Wisconsin Press, 1989.

Dromgoole, J. P. *Dr. Dromgoole's Yellow Fever: Heroes, Honors, and Horrors of 1878.* Louisville: John P. Morton, 1879.

DuBois, W. E. B. *Black Reconstruction.* New York: Harcourt Brace, 1935.

Duffy, John. *From Humors to Medical Science: A History of American Medicine.* Urbana: University of Illinois Press, 1993.

———. *The Sanitarians: A History of American Public Health.* Chicago: University of Illinois Press, 1990.

———. *Sword of Pestilence: The New Orleans Yellow Fever Epidemic of 1853.* Baton Rouge: Louisiana State University Press, 1966.

———. "Yellow Fever in the Continental United States during the Nineteenth Century." *Bulletin of the New York Academy of Medicine* 44 (June 1968): 687–701.

Dunning, William A. *Reconstruction: Political and Economic 1865–1877.* New York: Harper and Brothers, 1907.

Ellington, Cleta. *Christ: The Living Water; The Catholic Church in Mississippi.* Jackson, Miss.: Mississippi Today, 1989.

Ellis, John H. *Yellow Fever and Public Health in the New South.* Lexington: University Press of Kentucky, 1992.

Etheridge, Elizabeth W. *The Butterfly Caste: A Social History of Pellagra in the South.* Westport, Conn.: Greenwood, 1972.

Everman, Grace G., and Lavinia D. Fort. *History of St. James' Church, Greenville, Mississippi, 1869–1946.* Greenville, Miss.: Office Supply Company, 1946.

Falls, W. H. "Yellow Fever Treatments." *Cincinnati Lancet and Clinic* 1 (1878): 225–30.

Fant, John C., and Mabel B. Fant. *History of Mississippi: A School Reader.* Jackson: Mississippi Publishing Company, 1925.

Faust, Drew Gilpin. *Mothers of Invention: Women of the Slaveholding South in the American Civil War.* Chapel Hill: University of North Carolina Press, 1996.

Federal Writers' Project of the Works Progress Administration. *Mississippi: A Guide to the Magnolia State.* New York: Viking Press, 1938.

Foner, Eric. *Reconstruction: America's Unfinished Revolution, 1863–1877.* New York: Harper and Row, 1988.

Foner, Eric, and Olivia Mahoney. *America's Reconstruction: People and Politics after the Civil War.* Baton Rouge: Louisiana State University Press, 1997.

Foster, Gaines M. *Ghosts of the Confederacy: Defeat, the Lost Cause, and the Emergence of the New South, 1865–1913.* New York: Oxford University Press, 1987.

Franklin, John Hope. *Reconstruction after the Civil War.* Chicago: University of Chicago Press, 1960.

Gallagher, Gary W., and Alan T. Nolan, eds. *The Myth of the Lost Cause and Civil War History.* Bloomington: Indiana University Press, 2000.

Gant, Harris Allen. "The Epidemic at Water Valley, 1878." *Report of the Mississippi State Board of Health for the Years 1878–'79,* 69–72. Jackson, Miss.: Power and Barksdale, 1879.

———. "Yellow Fever in Mississippi, 1878–1905: Personal Recollections, Experiences, Reminiscences, Autobiography and History." *Mississippi Doctor* 13 (1936–37): 18–35.

Garner, James Wilford. *Reconstruction in Mississippi.* Gloucester, Mass.: Macmillan, 1901.

Gazzo, John B. C. *Yellow Fever Facts, as to Its Nature, Prevention and Treatment.* New Orleans: M. F. Dunn, 1878.

Gillson, Gordon E. "The Louisiana State Board of Health: The Formative Years." Ph.D. diss., Louisiana State University, 1960.

Gordon, T. H. "The Epidemic in Tillatoba and Vicinity, 1878." *Report of the Mississippi State Board of Health for the Years 1878–'79,* 79–82. Jackson, Miss.: Power and Barksdale, 1879.

Griffin, P. H. "Epidemic at Meridian, 1878." *Report of the Mississippi State Board of Health for the Years 1878–'79,* 155–59. Jackson, Miss.: Power and Barksdale, 1879.

Haley, J. Evetts. "Texas Fever and the Winchester Quarantine." *Panhandle-Plains Historical Review* 8 (1935): 37–53.

Haller, John S., Jr. *Medical Protestants: The Eclectics in American Medicine, 1825–1939.* Carbondale: Southern Illinois University Press, 1994.

Hamilton, William Baskerville. "Holly Springs, Mississippi, to the Year 1878." Master's thesis, University of Mississippi, 1931.

Hardenstein, Earnest. *The Yellow Fever Epidemic of 1878 and Its Homeopathic Treatment.* New Orleans: J. S. Rivers, 1879.

Harris, William C. *The Day of the Carpetbagger: Republican Reconstruction in Mississippi.* Baton Rouge: Louisiana State University Press, 1979.

———. "Formulation of the First Mississippi Plan: The Black Code of 1865." *Journal of Mississippi History* 29 (August 1967): 181–201.

———. *Presidential Reconstruction in Mississippi.* Baton Rouge: Louisiana State University Press, 1967.

———. "The Reconstruction of the Commonwealth, 1865–1870." In *A History of Mississippi,* vol. 1, ed. Richard Aubrey McLemore, 542–70. Jackson: University and College Press of Mississippi, 1973.

Harrison, James L., comp. *Biographical Directory of the American Congress, 1774–1949: The Continental Congress, September 5, 1774 to October 21, 1788 and the Congress of the United States, from the First to the Eightieth Congress, March 4, 1789 to January 3, 1949.* Washington, D.C.: Government Printing Office, 1949.

Hassler, Warren W., Jr. *General George B. McClellan: Shield of the Union.* Baton Rouge: Louisiana State University Press, 1957.

Headley, Katie McCaleb. *Claiborne County, Mississippi: The Promised Land.* Port Gibson, Miss.: Claiborne County Historical Society, 1976.

Hemphill, Marie M. *Fevers, Floods, and Faith: A History of Sunflower County, Mississippi, 1844–1976.* Indianola, Miss.: Sunflower County Historical Society, 1980.

Hildreth, Peggy Bassett. "Early Red Cross: The Howard Association of New Orleans, 1837–1878." *Louisiana History* 20 (Winter 1979): 49–75.

History of Marshall County, Mississippi: A Souvenir Edition Commemorating the Marshall County Centennial Celebration. Holly Springs, Miss.: Garden Club of Marshall County, 1936.

Holliday, D. C. "Remarks of Dr. D. C. Holliday, of New Orleans, on Yellow Fever, Made before the Baltimore Academy of Medicine, at a Special Meeting Held November 26th, 1878." *Maryland Medical Journal* 4 (1879): 207.

Holy Bible. Masonic ed. Wichita, Kans.: Heirloom, 1988.

Horsman, Reginald. *Josiah Nott of Mobile: Southerner, Physician, and Racial Theorist.* Baton Rouge: Louisiana State University Press, 1987.

Howell, Walter G. "The French Period: 1699–1763." In *A History of Mississippi,* vol. 1, ed. Richard Aubrey McLemore, 110–33. Jackson: University and College Press of Mississippi, 1973.

Humphreys, Margaret. *Yellow Fever and the South.* New Brunswick, N.J.: Rutgers University Press, 1992.

Hyman, Michael R. *The Anti-Redeemers: Hill-Country Political Dissenters in the Lower South from Redemption to Populism*. Baton Rouge: Louisiana State University Press, 1990.

In Memoriam: James Busby Norris, M.D. Chattanooga: Crandall, 1879.

Jones, Joseph. "Yellow Fever Epidemic of 1878 in New Orleans." *New Orleans Medical and Surgical Journal* 6 (February 1879): 605–7.

Kaufman, Martin. *Homeopathy in America: The Rise and Fall of a Medical Heresy*. Baltimore: Johns Hopkins University Press, 1971.

Keating, Bern. *A History of Washington County, Mississippi*. Greenville, Miss.: Greenville Junior Auxiliary, 1976.

Keating, J. M. *A History of the Yellow Fever: The Yellow Fever Epidemic of 1878 in Memphis, Tenn.* Memphis: Howard Association, 1879.

Kilpatrick, Andrew R. "An Account of the Yellow Fever Which Prevailed in Woodville, Mississippi in the Year 1844." *New Orleans Medical Journal* 2 (July 1845): 42.

King, Edward. *The Great South*, ed. W. Magruder Drake and Robert R. Jones. 1879. Baton Rouge: Louisiana State University Press, 1972.

Kiple, Kenneth F., and Virginia Himmelsteib King. *Another Dimension to the Black Diaspora: Diet, Disease, and Racism*. New York: Cambridge University Press, 1981.

Klein, Maury. *History of the Louisville and Nashville Railroad*. New York: Macmillan, 1972.

Kraut, Alan M. *Goldberger's War: The Life and Work of a Public Health Crusader*. New York: Hill and Wang, 2003.

Lawrence, Lulu Hayes. "Three by the Name of Jefferson Davis." *Confederate Veteran* 17 (November 1909): 533–35.

Laws of the State of Mississippi, Passed at a Regular Session of the Mississippi Legislature, Held in the City of Jackson, Commencing Jan. 8th, 1878, and Ending March 5th, 1878. Jackson, Miss.: Power and Barksdale, 1878.

Leavell, Z. T. *Baptist Annals, or Twenty-two Years with Mississippi Baptists: 1877–1899*. Philadelphia: American Baptist Publication Society, 1899.

Legan, Marshall Scott. "Mississippi and the Yellow Fever Epidemics of 1878–1879." *Journal of Mississippi History* 23 (August 1971): 199–217.

Livingston, J. *The Cause of and Remedy for Yellow Fever, as Explained in a Few Articles Published in the Daily City Item*. New Orleans: A. W. Hyatt, 1879.

Loewen, James W. *The Mississippi Chinese: Between Black and White*. Cambridge: Harvard University Press, 1971.

Loewen, James W., and Charles Sallis, eds. *Mississippi Conflict and Change*. New York: Pantheon Books, 1974.

Long, Alice S. "'My Dear, Manly Son': The Death of Jefferson Davis, Jr. at Buntyn Station, Tennessee, 1878." Master's thesis, University of Memphis, 1995.

Lord, Bob. "The Yellow Fever Epidemic of 1878 in Greenville." Greenville, Miss.: Washington County Historical Society, 1979.

Lowery, Robert, and William H. McCardle. *A History of Mississippi, from the Discovery of the Great River by Hernando DeSoto, Including the Earliest Settlement Made by the French, under Iberville, to the Death of Jefferson Davis.* Jackson, Miss.: R. H. Henry, 1891.

Martling, James A. "The Yellow Fever—1878." In *Poems of Home and Country,* 555–58. Boston: James H. Earle, 1885.

Mayes, Edward. "Charles Betts Galloway." *Publications of the Mississippi Historical Society* 11 (1910): 21–30.

McAlexander, Hubert Horton. *The Prodigal Daughter: A Biography of Sherwood Bonner.* Baton Rouge: Louisiana State University Press, 1981.

McClellan, George Brinton. *McClellan's Own Story: The War for the Union, the Soldiers Who Fought It, and the Civilians Who Directed It and His Relations to It and to Them.* New York: C. L. Webster, 1887.

McMillen, Neil. *Dark Journey: Black Mississippians in the Age of Jim Crow.* Urbana: University of Illinois Press, 1989.

McNeill, William H. *Plagues and Peoples.* New York: Anchor Press/Doubleday, 1976.

Medical and Surgical Directory of the Homeopathic Physicians of the United States and Canada. New York: A. L. Chatterton, 1897.

Mississippi Statistical Summary of Population, 1800–1960. Jackson: Mississippi Power and Light, 1962.

Monette, John Wesley. *Observations on the Epidemic Yellow Fever of Natchez and the South-west.* Louisville: Prentice and Weissinger, 1842.

North American Homeopathic Directory for 1877–78. Cleveland: Robison, Savage, 1878.

Numbers, Ronald L., and Todd L. Savitt, eds. *Science and Medicine in the Old South.* Baton Rouge: Louisiana State University Press, 1989.

Oakes, Sister Mary Paulinus. *Angels of Mercy: An Eyewitness Account of Civil War and Yellow Fever by a Sister of Mercy: A Primary Source.* Baltimore: Cathedral Foundation Press, 1998.

Ownby, Ted. *American Dreams in Mississippi: Consumers, Poverty, and Culture, 1830–1998.* Chapel Hill: University of North Carolina Press, 1999.

Parkes, Henry Bamford. *A History of Mexico.* Boston: Houghton Mifflin, 1969.

Patrick, Rembert. *The Reconstruction of the Nation.* New York: Oxford University Press, 1967.

Perman, Michael. "Counter Reconstruction: The Role of Violence in Southern

Redemption." In *The Facts of Reconstruction: Essays in Honor of John Hope Franklin,* ed. Eric Anderson and Alfred A. Moss Jr., 121–40. Baton Rouge: Louisiana State University Press, 1991.

Pillar, James J. "Religious and Cultural Life, 1817–1860." In *A History of Mississippi,* vol. 1, ed. Richard Aubrey McLemore, 378–419. Jackson: University and College Press of Mississippi, 1973.

Powell, J. H. *Bring Out Your Dead: The Great Plague of Yellow Fever in Philadelphia in 1793.* Philadelphia: University of Pennsylvania Press, 1949.

Power, J. L. *The Epidemic of 1878 in Mississippi: Report of the Yellow Fever Relief Work through J. L. Power, Grand Secretary of Masons and Grand Treasurer of Odd Fellows.* Jackson, Miss.: Clarion-Steam, 1879.

Pruitt, Olga Reed. *It Happened Here: True Stories of Holly Springs.* Holly Springs, Miss.: Marshall County Historical Society, 1950.

Quan, Robert Seto. *Lotus among the Magnolias: The Mississippi Chinese.* Jackson: University Press of Mississippi, 1982.

Ragland, Mary Lois, and Kathy Ragland Renfroe, comps. *Yellow Fever Epidemic of 1878.* Vicksburg, Miss.: n.p., 1987.

Ray, H. J. "The Epidemic in Grenada, 1878." *Report of the Mississippi State Board of Health for the Years 1878–'79,* 40–46. Jackson, Miss.: Power and Barksdale, 1879.

Report of the Executive Committee of the Yellow Fever National Relief Commission Organized at Washington, D.C., September 11, 1878, With Accompanying Reports of the Operations of the Relief Boat John M. Chambers, Receipts, Disbursements, Etc. Washington, D.C.: Government Printing Office, 1879.

Report of the Mississippi State Board of Health for the Years 1878–'79. Jackson, Miss.: Power and Barksdale, 1879.

Revels, James G. "Redeemers, Rednecks and Racial Integrity." In *A History of Mississippi,* vol. 1, ed. Richard Aubrey McLemore, 590–621. Jackson: University and College Press of Mississippi, 1973.

Riggs, Marvin A. "Some Aspects of the Administration of Governor John Marshall Stone of Mississippi." M.A. thesis, University of Alabama, 1947.

Ristic, Miodrag, and Julius P. Kreier. *Babesiosis.* New York: Academic, 1981.

Ritchie, John W. *Primer of Sanitation, Being a Simple Textbook on Disease Germs and How to Fight Them.* Yonkers-on-Hudson, N.Y.: World Book Company, 1913.

Roberts, Walter Adolphe. *Lake Pontchartrain.* New York: Bobbs-Merrill, 1943.

Rosenberg, Charles E. *The Cholera Years: The United States in 1832, 1849, and 1866.* 1962. Chicago: University of Chicago Press, 1987.

———. *Explaining Epidemics and Other Studies in the History of Medicine.* New York: Cambridge University Press, 1992.

Rousey, Dennis C. "Yellow Fever and Black Policemen in Memphis: A Post-Reconstruction Anomaly." *Journal of Southern History* 51 (August 1985): 357–74.

Sabin, Linda E. *Struggles and Triumphs: The Story of Mississippi Nurses, 1800–1950.* Jackson, Miss.: MHA Health, Research and Educational Foundation, 1998.

———. "Unheralded Nurses: Male Caregivers in the Nineteenth-Century South." In *Nurses' Work: Issues across Time and Place,* ed. Patricia D'Antonio et al., 49–64. New York: Springer, 2007.

Sansing, David G. "Congressional Reconstruction." In *A History of Mississippi,* vol. 1, ed. Richard Aubrey McLemore, 571–89. Jackson: University and College Press of Mississippi, 1973.

Savitt, Todd L. "Slave Health and Southern Distinctiveness." In *Disease and Distinctiveness in the American South,* ed. Todd L. Savitt and James Harvey Young, 120–53. Knoxville: University of Tennessee Press, 1988.

Savitt, Todd L., and James Harvey Young, eds. *Disease and Distinctiveness in the American South.* Knoxville: University of Tennessee Press, 1988.

Schmidt, H. D. "On the Nature of the Poison of Yellow Fever, and Its Prevention." *New York Medical Journal* 29 (May 1879): 449–84.

Semmes, A. T. "The Epidemic at Canton, 1878." *Report of the Mississippi State Board of Health for the Years 1878–'79,* 47–55. Jackson, Miss.: Power and Barksdale, 1879.

Shaplen, Robert. *Toward the Well-being of Mankind: Fifty Years of the Rockefeller Foundation.* Garden City, N.Y.: Doubleday, 1964.

Simkins, Francis Butler. *A History of the South.* New York: Knopf, 1953.

Slave Narratives: A Folk History of Slavery in the United States from Interviews with Former Slaves. The Federal Writers' Project of the Works Progress Administration for the States of Maryland and Mississippi. Vol. 9. Washington, D.C., 1941.

Smith, Ashbel, M.D., A.M. *Yellow Fever in Galveston, Republic of Texas, 1839: An Account of the Great Epidemic, Reprinted Together with a Biographical Sketch by Chauncey D. Lecke and Stories of the Men Who Conquered Yellow Fever.* 1839. Austin: University of Texas Press, 1951.

Spinzig, Charles. *Yellow Fever; Nature and Epidemic Character Caused by Meteorological Influences Verifies by the Epidemics of Shreveport and Memphis in 1873, By that of Savannah in 1876, By the Great Epidemic of the Mississippi Valley In 1878, And (In The Appendix) By The One of Memphis in 1879.* New York: Appleton, 1880.

Stampp, Kenneth M. *The Era of Reconstruction, 1865–1877.* New York: Vintage Books, 1965.

Sterling, Dorothy. *Black Foremothers: Three Lives.* New York: Feminist Press, 1988.

Stone, C. H. *History of the Mild Yellow Fever: Natchez, 1848.* Vidalia, La.: Concordia Intelligencer Office, 1849.

Strode, George E., ed. *Yellow Fever.* New York: McGraw Hill, 1951.

Strode, Hudson, ed. *Jefferson Davis' Private Letters, 1823–1889.* New York: Harcourt, Brace and World, 1966.

Sullivan, Charles L., and Murella Hebert Powell. *The Mississippi Gulf Coast: Portrait of a People.* Northridge, Calif.: Windsor, 1985.

Summers, Thomas O. *Yellow Fever.* Nashville: Wheeler Brothers, 1879.

Sumners, Cecil L. *The Governors of Mississippi.* Gretna, La.: Pelican, 1980.

Tenth Census of the United States, 1880: Population. Washington, D.C.: Government Printing Office, 1882.

Thomas, Hugh. *Cuba: The Pursuit of Freedom.* New York: Harper and Row, 1971.

Thomson, Samuel. *New Guide to Health; or, Botanic Family Physician.* Boston: J. Q. Adams, 1835.

Toner, John M. "Boards of Health in the United States." American Public Health Association, *Public Health Papers and Reports* 1 (1973): 499–521.

Toombs, R. S. "The Epidemic at Greenville, 1878." *Report of the Mississippi State Board of Health for the Years 1878–'79,* 63–65. Jackson, Miss.: Power and Barksdale, 1879.

Uhler, J. R. "The Prevention of Yellow Fever." *Maryland Medical Journal* 4 (November 1878): 10–11.

Underwood, Felix J., and R. N. Whitfield. *A Brief History of Public Health and Medical Licensure: State of Mississippi, 1799–1930.* Jackson: Mississippi State Board of Health, n.d.

U.S. Department of Agriculture. *Cotton and Cottonseed: Acreage, Yield, Production, Disposition, Price, Value By States, 1866–1952.* Washington, D.C.: Government Printing Office, 1955.

Wakelyn, Jon L. *Biographical Dictionary of the Confederacy.* Westport, Conn.: Greenwood Press, 1977.

Walker, F. A. *Tenth Census Report of the Productions of Agriculture.* Washington, D.C.: Government Printing Office, 1880.

Wall, E. G. *The State of Mississippi: Resources, Condition of Wants.* Jackson, Miss.: Clarion Steam Printing, 1879.

Warner, Margaret. "Local Control versus National Interest: The Debate over Southern Public Health, 1878–1884." *Journal of Southern History* 50 (August 1984): 407–28.

Warren, Andrew J. "Landmarks in the Conquest of Yellow Fever." In *Yellow Fever,* ed. George K. Strode, 5–37. New York: McGraw Hill, 1951.

Wells, Ida B. *Crusade for Justice: The Autobiography of Ida B. Wells,* ed. Alfreda M. Duster. Chicago: University of Chicago Press, 1970.

Wharton, R. G. "The Epidemic at Port Gibson, 1878." *Mississippi Board of Health Report for 1878–'79,* 66–69. Jackson, Miss.: Power and Barksdale, 1879.

Wharton, Vernon Lane. *The Negro in Mississippi, 1865–1890.* Chapel Hill: University of North Carolina Press, 1947.

White, William W. "Mississippi Confederate Veterans in Public Office, 1875–1890." *Journal of Mississippi History* 20 (January–October 1958): 147–55.

Williams, Greer. *The Plague Killers.* New York: Scribner, 1969.

Williams, James Levon, Jr. "Civil War and Reconstruction in the Yazoo Mississippi Delta, 1863–1875." Ph.D. diss., University of Arizona, 1992.

Wiltshire, Betty Couch, comp. *Mississippi Newspaper Abstracts.* 2 vols. Bowie, Md.: Heritage, 1987.

Woodworth, J. M. "Medical News." *Cincinnati Lancet and Clinic* 1 (1878): 160.

Zinn, Howard. *A People's History of the United States.* New York: HarperCollins, 1980.

Index

Aid Societies, African-American, 67–68, 71–72

Alcorn, James L., 3

Allopathic Medicine: definition of, 9–10; treatments, 15

American Medical Association, 15

American Public Health Association, 128, 129, 130

Andrews, W. H., 104

Archer, Stevenson, 62, 74, 104

Archer, W. B., 81

Bath, W. R., 63–64

Bay St. Louis, 36–37, 81, 95, 115

Beauvoir. *See* Davis, Jefferson, Sr.

Becton, J. E., 55

Beechland, ix

Ben Allen, 81

Benner, Hiram H., 103, 107

Billings, John Shaw, 127–130

Biloxi, 28, 40, 115

Black, Benjamin, 67

Broadwaters, Thomas M., 106

Brookhaven, 124

Buchanan, Victoria and George, 42

Buford, Mary and Albert, 34–36, 146n45

Cage, A. H., 113

Campbell, J. H., 70, 76, 77

Canton, 50, 71, 115, 134

Catholic Orphan Relief Association, 102

Claiborne County Board of Health, 33

Chunky (town), 98

Clark, John E., 24

Clinton, 29, 63

Coan, D. W., 76

Colored Preachers' Aid Society, 67–68

Columbus, 88

Committee for Orphans, 102

Compromise of 1877, 122

Compton, W. M., 113

Confederate Memorial Day, 97, 158n24

Cooper's Well, 29, 31, 145n32, 145n33

Cotton production, 104, 133–134

Cordwent, E., 104–105, 106

Crop-lien laws, 1

Cuba, Ten Year's War, 23

Cullom, Shelby M., 120

Davis, Jefferson, Jr., 96–97, 158n23, 158n24

Davis, Jefferson, Sr., 96–97, 116

Dennis, John L., 29–30, 145n33

Elections: 1868, 2; 1876, 4; 1878, 63

Elliott, Thomas, 24

Emily B. Souder, 23–24

Enforcement Act of 1871, 3

Eustis, James B., 130
Evarts, William H., 83

Fairchild, W. A., 64
Falconer, Kinloch, 59–60
Falls, W. H., 14
Featherstun, F. M., ix, 118–119
Finlay, Carlos, 111
Fraternal Order of the Masons, xi, 54
Friar's Point, 103, 115

Galloway, Charles Betts, 61
George, J. Z., 63
Germ theory, 111
Grand Gulf, 104
Green, Duncan C., 61–62
Greenville (town), 31, 74, 79–81, 104
Greenville Construction Company, 132–133
Greenville Quarantine Guards, 69
Greenwood (town): quarantine, 43;
    Greenville Times report, 155n22
Grenada County Board of Health, 77, 85
Grenada, 48–49, 55, 65–66, 75–78, 85, 88;
    African-American guard, 70; deaths
    in 1878, 154n11
Griffin, E. F., 37–38
Griffing, Cora, 29–30
Griffith, Benjamin Whitfield, 29–30

Haddick, H. T., 61
Hall, Charles S., 106
Handsboro, 28, 82–83, 87, 88, 115, 124;
    Handsboro Howards, 99–100
Hardenstein, A. O. H., 10–11, 14
Hardenstein, Earnest, 10, 99
Hardy, William H., 28
Harris, Isham G., 129
Harry, John J., 38
Hayes, Margaret and J. Addison, 96, 97
Hayes, Rutherford B., 103, 120, 122, 129, 130

Health Care Costs, 1878 epidemic, 134
Henderson, C. L., 22
Holland, W. J. L., 53, 97–98
Holly Springs, 41–43, 51–54, 60–61, 98,
    147n69, 147n70, 150n18; quarantines,
    22; Relief Committee, 51, 53, 56
Homeopathic Medicine: Samuel Chris-
    tian Hahnemann, 10; American Insti-
    tute of Homeopathy, 10, 15, 140n16,
    141n18; treatments of, 15
Howard Association, x, 33, 47, 51, 53,
    84–86, 99, 100, 102; John Howard,
    50; tributes to, 101, 142n38, 149n5,
    150n23
"Howards of the South, The" (poem),
    100–101
Hubbard, R. B., 120
Hughes, E. W., 113

Immigrants: Chinese, 69–70; deaths of,
    155n25
Iuka, 87

Jackson County Board of Health, 33
Jackson (town), 29, 68–69, 93–94, 114
John D. Porter, 27–28, 32
Johnston, Wirt, 26–27, 47, 131

Ku Klux Klan, xiv, 3, 55

Lake, 75, 153n6
Lamar, Lucius Q. C., 130
Leota Landing, 115
Littlepage, Ned, 63–64
Livingston, J., 14
Logtown, 60, 82
Longfellow, Henry Wadsworth, 57, 58,
    62, 98
Louisiana State Board of Health, xi–xii,
    20, 23
Loyal Leagues, 2, 58
Lyon, John E., 82, 95–96

Marshall, Charles Kimball, 61

McCallum, Mary and George C., 75

McClellan, George B., 120, 122

McCormick, P. J., 92

McDowell, Katharine Bonner (Sherwood Bonner), 57–58, 98, 150n30

McInnis, S. A., 37–38

McRae, J. D., 49

Mead, J. A., 30, 60

Meridian, 90–91; race riots, 3; quarantine, 22; aid society, 91; population of, 143n8; monetary relief to, 157n6

Mitchell, R. W., 110

Mississippi Black Code, xiii

Mississippi City, 28, 40, 95, 115

Mississippi College, 31

Mississippi Law Code: 1857, x; 1878, 144n22

Mississippi Plan, xiv

Mississippi Quarantine Act, 38

Mississippi River Flood (1874), 105

Mississippi State Board of Health, ix, 25–26, 34, 45, 47, 48, 111–114, 126, 131; members deaths in 1878, 113; investigative meeting in 1879, 161n7

Mitchell, R. W., 13

Monetary aid, 83–84, 119, 124

Moseley, Robert J., 91

Moss Point, 124

Mulatto Bayou, 95

Murphy, Emma and John, 96

Natchez: Jewish citizens, 46; quarantine, 87–88

National Board of Health, 114, 127

New South, 130, 151n39, 155n20, 160n45

Newton (town), 105

Nicholson, George, 30

Nursing: 33, 64–65, 54–55, 101–102, 149n13; Howard nurses, 50; Catholic nursing orders, 50, 53; African–American women, 64–65; male nurses, 152n56, 152n58, 152n59

Oberti, Father Anacletus, 52–53, 149n12

Ocean Springs, 22, 95, 115

Order of Freemasons, 50, 90, 91, 99, 100, 102, 123

Order of Sisters of Charity, 49–50, 52–53, 66, 92, 96, 149n13, 149n15

Osyka, 116–117

Page, Tillman, 62

Pascagoula, 28, 94, 100; fundraiser, 84, 156n37; Patrick Mullett obituary, 157n14

Pass Christian, 75, 81–82, 115, 117

Patton, Buck, 93

Peabody Association: Vicksburg organization, 106–107; New Orleans organization, 160n46, 160n47

Pearlington, 30, 95

Pearl River, 39–40

Pearson, Henry Hume, 78, 154n16

Pelaez, Charles, 30–31

Poleicho, Mateo, 82

Port Gibson, 31, 32, 78–79, 87, 104

Power, J. L., 50, 76, 90, 100, 116–117, 122

Public Health: weakness, 64; movement, 113, 123, 126; McGowan Bill, 130

Quarantine: failure, 31, 32, 92, 116; "Six Sisters," 39–40; federal quarantine law, 130–131

Race relations, 62–68, 69, 70–71, 104–106, 134–135

Railroads: prior to Civil War, 21; post-Civil War, 21–22; The New Orleans and Mobile, 30, 132; Chicago, St. Louis & New Orleans, 44, 45, 131–132, 134; Illinois Central, 44; Alabama Great Southern, 65; Greenville, Co-

lumbus and Birmingham, 74; Vicks-
burg and Meridian, 75; Memphis and
Charleston, 97
Rattlesnake Bayou, 81
Reed, Bob, 65–66
Relief Efforts: African-American, 71;
Jewish, 102; U.S. government, 102;
John M. Chambers relief boat, 102–
104, 109, 159n38
Rice, C. A., 122
Rivinac, Peter, 107
Rockefeller Foundation, 136
Rockwood, W. M., 64

Scranton, 37, 94
Sectional Healing, 86, 99, 135; governors'
Thanksgiving Proclamations, 120–122
Semmes, A. T., 134
Senate Resolution 1462, 130
Sharecropping, 1, 63, 138n2
Shaw University, 58
Shepherd, Alexander R. *See* Yellow Fever
National Relief Commission
Shreve, Charles, 78
Sisters of Mercy, 52, 98, 158n26
Sisters of the Holy Family, 68
St. Mary's Convent. *See* Order of Sisters
of Charity
Stith, George W., 106
Stone, John M., 4–5, 46–47, 84, 139n15
Stoneville, 74
Stonewall (town), 40–41, 101

Terrene (town), 103–104
Thomson, Samuel: early life, 11–12;
botanico-medical system, 12; treat-
ments, 15
Trigg, A. B., 81
Trigg, Nancy Hurst, 62

Uhler, J. R., 110
United States Public Health Service,
136
University of Mississippi, 31

Vance, Z. B., 54
Vicksburg, 1, 3–4, 31, 33–34, 63, 73–74,
79, 86–87, 98–99, 102, 104, 114, 124–
125; Frank J. Fisher Funeral Home,
73, 144n28, 153n1; population of,
143n8, 162n14; Civil War, 155n18;
physician deaths, 156n41; Ashbury
Cemetery, 159n27

Water Valley, 43–45, 55–56, 123
Wells, Ida Bell, 58–59, 151n35
Whitehead, P. F., 113
Woodworth, John M., 127–130, 164n14

Yalobusha County Board of Health, 45
Yandell, L. P., 110
Yarborough, J. S. 75
Yazoo City, 91–92, 115, 124
Yellow Fever National Relief Commission, 103, 127, 129, 163n4
Yellow fever: description, 6, 140n4, 161n4;
origin, 6–7, 137n5, 139n2, 142n42,
143n12; symptoms/treatments, 7–9,
12–15, 113, 140n14, 141n32; 141n34;
miasmic theory, 15–16, 33–34; fomite
theory, 16, 35, 69, 80, 142n39; social causation, 16–17; 1853 epidemic,
19–20; 1853 quarantine, 21; Nicholson pavement, 110; Mississippi deaths
in 1878, 117, 126, 148n81, 163n4; New
Orleans deaths in 1878, 126; Memphis deaths in 1878, 126; monetary
costs of, 134; total deaths in 1878 epidemic, 163n4